Overview of the Book

Pocket Atlas of Endodontics

Rudolf Beer, D.D.S, Ph.D.
Private Dental Practioner
Essen, Germany

Andrej M. Kielbassa, M.D.
Professor, Charité Berlin
Benjamin Franklin Campus
Department of Operative Dentistry
and Periodontology
Berlin, Germany

Michael A. Baumann, D.D.S.,
Ph.D.
Certified Specialist and
Member of the European
Society of Endodontology (ESE)
Department of Operative
Dentistry and Periodontology
Dental School, University of Cologne
Cologne, Germany

Translated by Thomas M. Hassell, D.D.S., Ph.D.

780 illustrations

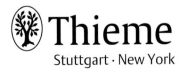

Thieme
Stuttgart · New York

Library of Congress Cataloging-in-Publication Data

Beer, R. (Rudolf)
[Taschenatlas der Endodontie. English]
Pocket atlas of endodontology / Rudolf Beer, Michael A. Baumann, Andrej M. Kielbassa; translated by Thomas M. Hassell.
p. ; cm.
Includes index.
ISBN 3-13-139781-0 (GTV : alk. paper) –
ISBN 1-58890-347-8 (TNY : alk. paper)
1. Endodontics–Atlases.
2. Endodontics–Handbooks, manuals, etc.
3. Root canal therapy–Atlases.
I. Baumann, Michael A.
II. Kielbassa, Andrej M.
III. Title.
[DNLM: 1. Dental Pulp Diseases–Handbooks.
2. Root Canal Therapy–Handbooks.
WU 49 B414t 2006a]
RK351.B445 2006
617.6'342'00222–dc22   2005022859

This book is an authorized and revised translation of the German edition published and copyrighted 2004 by Georg Thieme Verlag, Stuttgart, Germany. Title of the German edition: Taschenatlas der Endodontie.

Translator: Thomas M. Hassell, DDS, PhD, Flagstaff, Arizona, USA

Illustrator: Albert Ruech, Spay, Germany

© 2006 Georg Thieme Verlag,
Rüdigerstrasse 14, 70469 Stuttgart, Germany
http://www.thieme.de
Thieme New York, 333 Seventh Avenue,
New York, NY 10001 USA
http://www.thieme.com

Typesetting by OADF, www.oadf.de
Printed in Germany by Appl, Wemding
ISBN 3-13-139781-0 (GTV)
ISBN 1-58890-347-8 (TNY)   1 2 3 4 5 6

Important note: Medicine is an ever-changing science undergoing continual development. Research and clinical experience are continually expanding our knowledge, in particular our knowledge of proper treatment and drug therapy. Insofar as this book mentions any dosage or application, readers may rest assured that the authors, editors, and publishers have made every effort to ensure that such references are in accordance with **the state of knowledge at the time of production of the book**.

Nevertheless, this does not involve, imply, or express any guarantee or responsibility on the part of the publishers in respect to any dosage instructions and forms of applications stated in the book. **Every user is requested to examine carefully** the manufacturers' leaflets accompanying each drug and to check, if necessary in consultation with a physician or specialist, whether the dosage schedules mentioned therein or the contraindications stated by the manufacturers differ from the statements made in the present book. Such examination is particularly important with drugs that are either rarely used or have been newly released on the market. Every dosage schedule or every form of application used is entirely at the user's own risk and responsibility. The authors and publishers request every user to report to the publishers any discrepancies or inaccuracies noticed. If errors in this work are found after publication, errata will be posted at www.thieme.com on the product description page.

Special thanks to my wife, Marianne,
whose input and support tremendously
influenced the successful completion of this book.

Rudolf Beer

I dedicate this book to my parents,
for their loving and constant support
of my education and my choices in life.

Michael A. Baumann

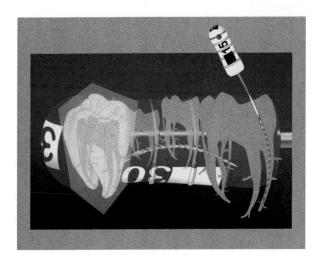

Preface

For many decades, the dental specialty of endodontics was a satisfactorily stable, if somewhat static, profession. However, recent years have witnessed dramatic progress in the discipline. A perfect example of this can be found in the fact that our book *Endodontology*, published almost seven years ago, was followed only one year later by a new volume that reported rapid development in the clinical discipline, especially the remarkable developments with nickel-titanium (NiTi) files. In addition, our original book only *hinted* at new possibilities in endodontics offered by the surgical microscope, ultrasonic devices and microsurgery; in most recent years, these have become state-of-the-art in the daily practice of endodontics.

In the interim, actually within the most recent months, further developments and new procedures have emerged, and scientific studies have contributed significantly to improved understanding of the new instruments and new materials, including possibilities and limitations.

The introduction of high-tech equipment such as the surgical microscope, in combination with ultrasonic devices, makes possible today therapeutic endeavors and treatment successes that were virtually unattainable only a few years ago, and then only by a very small number of endodontic enthusiasts.

NiTi files utilized with special computer-controlled motors today permit predictably improved root canal instrumentation in virtually all cases. The significance of chemical adjuncts during canal irrigation has been re-emphasized. Also, the actual filling of the canal using softened gutta percha and a sealer has been perfected, leading to its much broader applicability. Emphasis has been placed, and new knowledge employed concerning not only the impermeable apical closure of the root canal system, but also the importance of an impermeable *coronal* seal, especially in terms of the ever-present danger of post-endodontic coronal leakage.

All of this new knowledge and all of these new materials and devices offer tremendous potential for endodontic successes. However, these also demand from the clinician a continually changing orientation, and an up-date of her/his knowledge, because while technical aids and new materials are important, the theoretical background and understanding/ knowledge of their clinical application is of even more significance. It is with these concepts and principles in mind that we offer this new, compact yet comprehensive book, which will provide a rapid and contemporary orientation in the daily dental/endodontic practice.

The half-life of knowledge today renders any attempt at printed fixation of new knowledge only a momentary endeavor. Modern media such as the internet and all of its possibilities for research present a primary option for each individual to achieve up-to-the-minute orientation world-wide. Nevertheless, in the future *books* will maintain their position on the front line because they offer information in an accessible and always available form, in black and white, for orientation and concentration.

Rudolf Beer, Essen
Michael A. Baumann, Cologne
Andrej M. Kielbassa, Berlin

Acknowledgments

The purpose of a "pocket atlas" is to provide visualization of important concepts in order to simplify understanding of such scientific concepts, and to render them accessible. We therefore thank Mr. A. Ruech (Spay) who created so many of our illustrations with full understanding of the discipline. The majority of the photographs of instruments was provided by Mr. S. Gutbier and T. Schöning (Photography Department, Dental School, University of Cologne). These individuals deserve our thanks, as well as Ms. S. Urbanek (MTA of the Department of Dentistry, University of Cologne), who provided several SEM photomicrographs, and Dr. G. Mayerhöfer (Düsseldorf) for the excellent prosthetic treatment of several of the patients depicted in this book.

From Thieme Medical Publishers, we authors continuously enjoyed unfailing support and truly excellent responses to any and all questions and situations, from Dr. Urbanowicz and Mr. M. Pohlmann.

A project as comprehensive as this *Pocket Atlas of Endodontics* receives its lifeblood from discussions and interactions with other authors and collaborators; therefore, we take this opportunity to thank all of our clinical colleagues who cannot be named in this short presentation, but who have contributed so valuably with tips and professional discussions, which led to the succesful conclusion of this work.

Any perfect transfer of ideas can occur only via an ideal format. The virtual creation of this book was substantially both understood and undertaken in so many aspects by the collaborators in the two firms listed below, to whom we express our sincere thanks:

• Dr. Sterckenburg and Dr. A. Guggenmos in the *Vereingte Dentalwerke München*

• Mr. Maillefer of the Swiss company *Maillefer Ballaigues*.

We are grateful to Dr. Thomas Hassell (Arizona, USA) for his competent Anglicization of our book, and Ms. Censeri Abare (Florida, USA) for her precision in preparing the English manuscript.

Finally our special thanks go to our former mentors, Professor Gängler, Professor Löst, Professor Ketterl and Professor Heilwig, who initially awakened our appreciation of endodontics and who guided us during our many years of scientific endeavors in this discipline.

Foreword

Throughout the decades of the late 1800s and throughout most of the early 1900s the dental specialty of endodontics was essentially stagnant: Dental caries led to pulpal involvement, inflammation and pain. In almost all patients, the "treatment of choice" was, simply, tooth extraction. However, patients with sufficient means were invited into the risky realm of "root canal treatment," which offered no guarantees of success and which was supported by only a paucity of clinical or scientific base. It was a purely mechanical effort to eliminate a patient's pain by removing the source of that pain, literally by removing the nerves within a tooth. No nerve – no pain! There was no scientific inquiry, no "differential diagnosis," only a tedious mechanical endeavor.

And then, in the middle of the 20th Century, innovative and targeted clinical (animal and human) as well as laboratory research by pioneers including Blaney, Grossman, Bender and Seltzer, and Schröder, and later Vertucci and Stashenko, provided endodontics with the scientific basis it had always lacked. Scientific and clinical findings spurred a virtual endodontic renaissance among dental practitioners. Such enthusiasm quickly spurred dental manufacturers to their own renaissance in materials and equipment targeted toward effective and long-term successful endodontic therapy.

This *Pocket Atlas of Endodontics* is a contemporary presentation of the state-of-the-art in root canal therapy. The book makes no claim to being the "final word" in the discipline; rather, it *objectively* presents where endodontics is today. It presents many approaches to the myriad of maladies of the endodontium, and presents the appropriate clinical and scientific evidence to support various treatment modalities. But the strength of this book is the authors' reluctance to endorse any single technique. The authors demand of the reader is that she/he draw her/his own conclusions relating to the treatment of various types of pulpal involvement. The authors openly and frankly acknowledge that clinical endeavors must be based upon scientific research, the knowledge that has emanated therefrom, each clinician's strengths, and above all, upon each patient's understanding of her/his affliction and each patient's desires for reconciliation of an uncomfortable situation.

This book provides almost astonishingly complete coverage of a rapidly-advancing medical/dental discipline, with a minimum of verbiage to confuse the practitioner or obfuscate the issue at hand. The illustrations are of high quality and reduced to the basics required for understanding a concept. This book addresses new and patient-centered exigencies directly and adroitly, presenting traditional endodontic concepts as well as surgical intervention in a new and refreshing light. This book addresses the *consequences* of endodontic treatment as well as the technical aspects of patient care in the daily practice of dentistry.

The authors have invested extensive time and effort to freshly describe the etiology and pathogenesis of various disorders of the endodontium, encompassing the most contemporary clinical and basic research findings. The literature citations are up-to-date, but limited to the most significant articles that relate to daily practice.

I am pleased and proud to introduce this new book, which effectively bridges the gap between scientific esoterica and the practitioner's daily need for relevant knowledge.

Thomas Hassell, Flagstaff, Arizona

Table of Contents

Disinfection of the Root Canal ... 152

Temporary Closure ... 174

Filling the Root Canal ... 176

The **endodontium** consists of mineralized (dentin) and nonmineralized (pulp) portions, and encompasses the functional-anatomic relationships of the dentin-pulp system.

The **dentin** consists of:

- odontoblasts and their processes
- dentinal tubules
- peritubular dentin
- intertubular dentin
- mantle dentin.

The **odontoblasts** are densely aligned along the inner surface of the dentin. Their processes extend through the entire dentin layer to the dentinoenamel junction, and are up to 5 mm long depending on the dentin thickness. The odontoblasts are interconnected through gap junctions as well as tight junctions. These cells synthesize the **primary dentin**, consisting of type I collagen, glycoproteins, and glycosaminoglycans. This organic precursor later becomes mineralized at some distance from the odontoblast layer.

The majority of the dentin is referred to **circumpulpal dentin** and is located between mantle dental and the pulp chamber. **Mineralization** begins only when the predentin has achieved a certain degree of histologic maturity.

The odontoblastic processes course within the dentinal tubules. Between the cytoplasmic membrane of the processes and the canal wall there is often a periodontoblastic space that contains tissue fluid and collagen fibrils, as well as dentin matrix.

The very densely mineralized **peritubular dentin** covers the dentin canal wall. It is not found in predentin. Its thickness depends on patient age, but it may also be laid down as a defense against external influences. Dentinal tubules with small lumens and thick peritubular walls appear as a translucent zone when viewed in ground sections under a light microscope; this zone is called **sclerosed dentin**.

The dentinal tubules are separated from each other by less densely mineralized **intertubular dentin**.

The peripheral layer of dentin exhibits highly branching odontoblastic processes referred to as **mantle dentin**. In contrast to the circumpulpal dentin, this layer is less densely mineralized. Dental enamel is attached to the mantle dentin. As demonstrated by R.M. Frank and coworkers, nerve fibers also extend to the dentinoenamel junction. Thus the vitality of dentin tissue is not the result of hydrodynamic transfer of irritation, as was long believed, but rather for the most part on direct nerve conduction, i.e., the nerve endings are directly stimulated.

The **pulp** consists of loose connective tissue. In addition to odontoblasts it contains fibroblasts, replacement cells, and defense cells. The **fibroblasts** represent the largest cell population, and appear as inactive and active cells, the latter producing the intercellular substance and collagen precursors. **Replacement cells** are undifferentiated mesenchymal cells that cannot be differentiated from fibroblasts by shape. These cells may replace odontoblasts as well as defense cells, and assume their functions.

Figures

A Structure of a secretory odontoblast.

B Formation of circumpulpal dentin: Predentin, secreted by odontoblasts, mineralizes at a distance ca. 20 µm distal to the odontoblasts, emanating from focal centers that accumulate as calcium globules (circles). These aggregate in the subsequent mineralization process. At this time, the formation of peritubular dentin begins.

C The formation of secondary as well as intertubular dentin (dark) reduces the size of the pulp chamber as well as the dentinal tubules (right).

D *Zone-like formation of the coronal pulp* from the odontoblastic zone (middle), subodontoblastic, cell-poor zone, and cell-rich bipolar zone (below). The latter is characterized by fibroblasts, undifferentiated replacement cells, and the Raschkow nerve plexus.

E The *Hertwig epithelial sheath* induces the differentiation of ectomesenchymal cells of the tooth bud into odontoblasts.

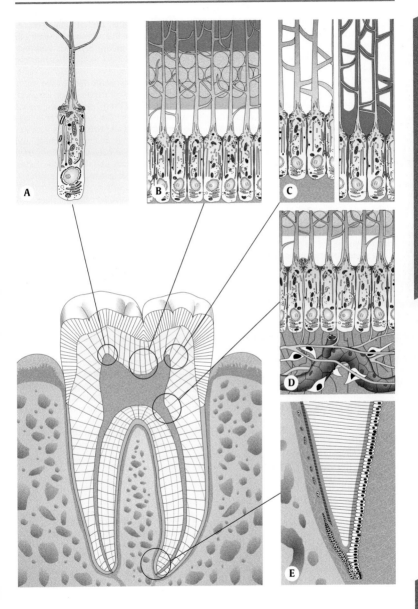

Enamel caries, clinically detectable as an opaque discoloration, is reversible. Initial caries is divided into **three zones**: On the advancing caries front, a translucent layer is visible; a dark zone is attached. The body of the lesion represents the third zone, suprajacent to the apparently intact enamel surface.

Dentin caries is differentiated into early and advanced lesions: In an **early dentin carious lesion** histologic changes occur without enamel cavitation, whereby plaque toxins diffuse through the enamel and cause secondary (reparative) dentin formation as well as early accumulations of inflammatory cells. If the cause is eliminated, partial regression of dentin caries can occur at this stage.

With **advanced dentin caries**, on the other hand, enamel cavitation has already occurred. The bacterial destruction expands along the mantle dentin. The lesion becomes more extensive, undermining the enamel. Initially, the advanced lesion is a combination of defense and destruction. Later in the process, there is unhindered penetration of bacteria. At this stage, **six zones** can be differentiated:

1 softening and liquefaction, with excavatable dentin
2 demineralization with multiple areas of destruction
3 advancing bacteria penetrate the dentinal tubuli
4 hypermineralization
5 the transparent zone is clinically hard
6 reparative (secondary) dentin forms on the pulpal wall.

Diagnosis

Clinical examination alone is not sufficient to determine the depth of the carious lesion in occlusal fissures. In a study by Tveit, teeth that were scored as noncarious clinically were examined histologically and only 10% were caries-free while 76% already exhibited enamel caries. Of 131 lesions with small occlusal cavitation, 41 already exhibited dentin caries, which had only been detected by clinical probing in 31 instances. In a study of the influence of clinical probing, in one group teeth were only examined visually, others with probing. One week later, the teeth were extracted. The histologic examination revealed only seven carious defects in the group without probing, but after clinical probing 60 defects of tooth hard structure were observed. In addition, in this group there was even evidence of tooth surface destruction into the dentin.

Radiographic diagnosis doubles the sensitivity for detection of fissure caries. However, more than half of even deeper dentin lesions remain undetected. The capability of detecting carious teeth (sensitivity) is 12% with visual diagnosis alone, 14% with probing, and 20% with the use of magnifying loupes. Only with the additional use of bitewing radiographs was it possible to increase the sensitivity to 49%.

In a study of proximal carious lesions, 66% exhibited opaque enamel discoloration, 32% of the teeth showed small lesions, and 1.3% pronounced cavitation. In teeth with a radiographic index of grade 1 (enamel), 13% exhibited clinical dentin caries, and with a radiographic index of 3, 58% exhibited cavitations. There was no direct correlation between radiographic findings and actual clinical observations. In the posterior arch segments, only 30% of carious lesions can be conclusively determined using bitewing radiographs. C4 lesions (deep dentin caries), however, can be precisely detected.

In almost every case, the histologic picture of caries is more advanced than what the radiograph shows. Experience and degree of training enhance caries diagnosis. Experienced practitioners interpret radiographs more cautiously. Dental students, on the other hand, too often diagnosis caries, with the danger of "overtreatment."

Histology

A/B Penetrating advanced dentin caries, with carious opening into the pulpal tissue and adjacent necrosis.

C/D Dilation of the dentinal tubules as ampullae and garlands (zones 1–3).

E/F Bacterial expansion of dentinal tubules.

G Bacteria can also penetrate into a tubular reparative dentin (zone 6).

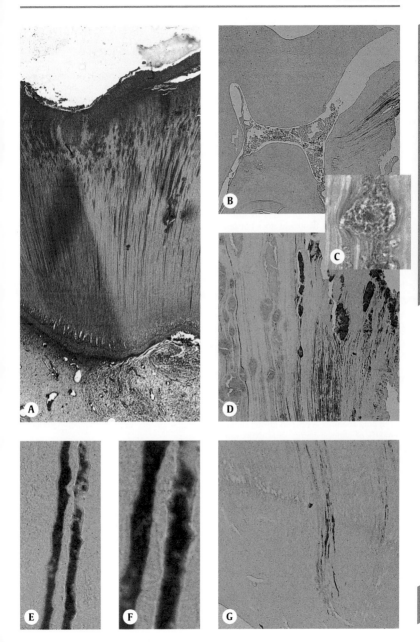

In the absence of any therapeutic measures, profound caries caused by infection will lead to an inflammatory host response within the pulp, and the ultimate consequence will be necrosis. The goal in tooth maintenance is therefore to completely remove all infected tooth substance. In this way, the further progress of toxins, antigens, and bacteria can be effectively inhibited. Use of special **color indicators** can significantly simplify such clinical treatment.

The cause of dental caries is bacterial infection. Since the spatial expanse of carious involvement cannot be absolutely determined, if any diseased tooth structure is left behind, more or less high concentrations of bacteria near the pulp can be expected. This sort of compromise during treatment does not provide true causal treatment of the infection.

Even if the number of remaining microorganisms can be significantly reduced following definitive treatment, there remains a long-term risk of remaining caries and the danger of pulpal involvement. Combating bacteria with topical medicaments (e.g., calcium hydroxide-based), even in the most optimum experimental conditions, does not lead to sterile relationships.

For this reason alone, the **removal of caries** must be complete, even when there is a danger of opening the pulp chamber. This is supported by the fact that the pulpal tissues are either acutely or chronically inflamed if the carious process has already reached the pulp. If the pulp chamber is opened during clinical removal of carious dentin, vital extirpation must be performed. If carious dentin is completely removed and the pulp is accidentally opened in an area of healthy dentin, direct pulp capping can be performed.

Following application of a caries detector solution, dentin caries exhibits a **distinctive red coloration**; in dentin regions very near the pulp, where a high number of dentinal tubules exist, a (reversible) pink color is characteristic, but this is not indicative of a carious process.

The effective, positive use of the caries detector was demonstrated in a long-term study of 224 cavities. Neither after one, nor after three years' observation was it possible to diagnosis any "recurrent caries." During examinations five to six years later, four carious lesions were detected beneath the restorations and three immediately adjacent to the restorations.

The stainability of carious dentin does not result from demineralization, but from the caries-induced alterations in collagen structure.

The removal of the stained dentin leads to complete elimination of bacteria. In some patients, the caries detector will reveal infected dentin beneath natural staining. In such cases, it is important to recognize that the lack of reaction by the pulp-dentin complex in nonvital teeth results in bacteria progressing uninhibited into the dentin.

With complete elimination of the infection, and because of minimum preparation trauma resulting from the selective carious removal, it is possible to reduce to a minimum any noxious effects on the pulpal tissues. In addition is the fact that the caries detector solution is harmless and aside from rare and minor pain sensation, it does not cause pulpal irritation during preparation.

The caries detector is a valuable aid for complete elimination of infection during treatment for caries. If endodontic intervention becomes unavoidable, the caries detector provides a valuable enhancement in keeping with accepted principles of asepsis.

Case Presentation

A Fissure with a localized breach; "hidden caries" in a vital tooth

B Corresponding radiographic picture

C Appearance before staining

D Staining of remaining caries

E Appearance after complete caries removal

F Conditioning of the tooth structures

G Definitive ceramic cusp replacement

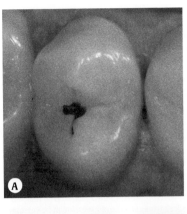

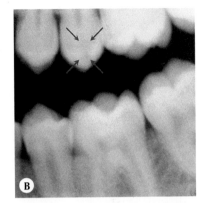

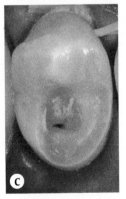

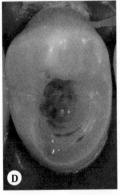

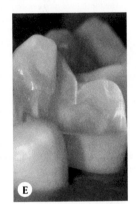

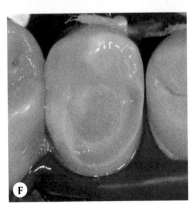

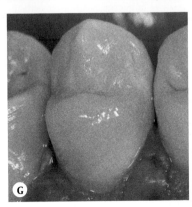

The pulp cannot be directly inspected or examined. Except for pain, all other symptoms of inflammation cannot be adjudged. In accordance with the reports by Baume and other authors, a **clinical classification of pulpal inflammation** has been presented as four groups: (1) asymptomatic and (2) symptomatic reversible inflammation, (3) irreversible phase, and (4) pulpal necrosis.

- **Asymptomatic pulp pathology** is painless. The tooth responds positively to a vitality/sensitivity test. The carious process may extend deeply into dentin, but not into the pulp.
- With **reversible pulpitis**, pain is elicited by cold, sweet, or sour and the carious process has not yet invaded the pulp. Percussion of the tooth is negative or inconclusive.
- With **irreversible pulpitis**, pain may occur spontaneously, and increase with heat. The percussion test is usually negative, but may be mildly positive.
- With **pulpal necrosis**, pain may be absent or may be extremely severe. The sensitivity test is negative or extremely positive and, in some patients, the radiograph may depict a periapical lesion.

Initial histologic manifestations of inflammatory reactions within the pulp occur during the **progression of enamel caries into dentin**. The odontoblastic processes end at the dentinoenamel junction in a layer of sclerosed dentin, where peritubular dentin is formed, followed by mineralization of the odontoblastic processes. At this site, numerous bacteria reside.

If the carious process is **superficial** and **chronic**, one notes formation of secondary dentin and mild inflammatory cell infiltration, in addition to reduction of the odontoblastic layer.

With **active caries**, on the other hand, there is a massive inflammatory cell infiltration with only minimal secondary dentin formation, in addition to pathologically altered odontoblasts. The lysosomal enzymes released by damaged neutrophilic granulocytes and macrophages lead to endothelial cell necrosis, and the consequence is increased vascular permeability and a resultant extracellular edema. At this stage of the carious

process, nerve fibers appear to be only relatively minimally damaged.

The area of inflammation expands, but is localized only to small foci within the coronal pulp, without endangering the remaining pulpal tissue. Pathologic mineralization along the canal wall, as well as initial denticle formation, may also occur.

During inflammation, endothelial cells within the blood vessels are activated to express adhesion molecules, which elevate the attachment of circulating leukocytes. This, and a slowed blood flow, permit the neutrophilic granulocytes to attach to the endothelium and extravasate into the neighboring pulpal tissues. Upon the surface receptors of macrophages, e.g., CD14, bacterial lipopolysaccharide (LPS) binds, which can be released within the dentinal tubuli upon death of gram-negative bacteria. This activates macrophages, which secrete cytokines and chemokines that enhance inflammation.

For example, the cytokine TNF-α can activate endothelial cells to release IgG and complement and activate leukocytes, which leads to extravascular edema and therefore to pain. IL-1 and IL-6 elicit lymphocyte activation and therefore elevated antibody production; IL-8 attracts neutrophilic granulocytes, basophiles, and T cells to the focus of infection, and IL-12 induces CD4 T-cells to TH1 cells.

Histology

A Secondary (repair) dentin and denticle formation adjacent to the advanced dentin caries.

B Secondary dentin has only few tubules and is bordered by few odontoblasts.

C Within the pulp horn, one notes an accumulation of inflammatory cells.

D/E Note the initial disintegration of the odontoblastic layer and the obvious inflammatory cell infiltration, without tissue necrosis.

F Bacteria infiltrate coronally into dentinal tubules. At the pulpal wall, neutrophilic granulocytes migrate toward adjacent tubule entrances and release tissue-destructive enzymes.

G Neutrophilic granulocytes, evident in the predentin layer and within dentinal tubules.

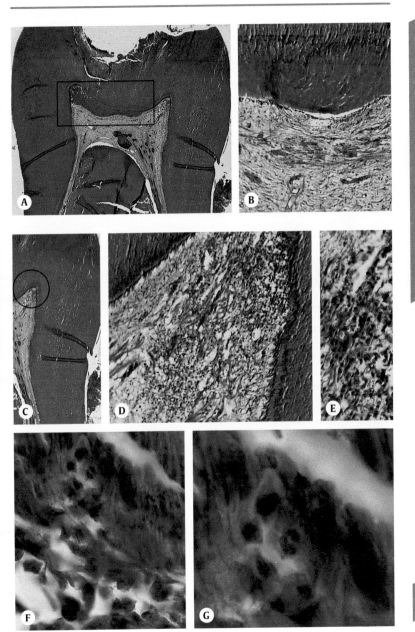

After bacteria invade into the dentinal tubules, **neutrophilic granulocytes** migrate in the direction of the tubule entrances near the pulp; there, the granulocytes die and release lysosomal enzymes that destroy pulpal tissue. During the subsequent phagocytosis of the destroyed tissue by polymorphonuclear or mononuclear phagocytes, the uptake of cellular debris leads to additional **release of lysosomal enzymes**, with subsequent tissue destruction and a chemotactic attraction for additional inflammatory cells.

The **offensive agents** that enhance the inflammatory reaction are bacteria and their metabolic and breakdown products, as well as the products of decomposition of the dentin itself. A **vicious circle** is initiated, which manifests itself as an irreversible pulpitis.

In areas near to the necrotic regions, the pulpal tissue becomes saturated with neutrophilic granulocytes, which phagocytize bacteria. This elicits the disintegration of large areas of the pulp; this process expands in an apical direction.

However, the histologic picture of an acute inflammation with prevalence of acute inflammatory cells does not necessarily mean that all clinical symptoms of acute inflammation will be present. In more than 25% of all cases of deep caries with partial pulpal necrosis and severe inflammation, no history of pain symptom is reported. The depth of the carious process also does *not* correlate with the occurrence of pain.

In cases of irreversible pulpitis with necrosis, there is almost always a widening of the apical periodontal ligament space. The etiology of this early periapical reaction appears to be toxin penetration through intact pulpal tissue. **Endotoxin**, released from the external membrane of gram-negative bacteria (LPS), can also elicit the complement reaction. **Complement activation** affects a release of biologically active peptides, the consequence of which is an increase in vascular permeability and attraction of neutrophilic granulocytes and macrophages. Lysosomal enzymes that are released during phagocytosis cause the actual tissue destruction. Small complement fragments, especially C5a, can induce local inflammation and intensify it. C5a also activates mast cells, mediators of histamine and TNF-α

release, all of which intensify the inflammation.

Tempering the **destructive effects** of the complement system and the rapid elevation of its activation by the enzyme cascade, there are also complement-regulating proteins that can inhibit excessive tissue destruction.

In sum, the complement system is one of the most important mechanisms through which pathogens are recognized and an effective defense against bacteria and their metabolic products is raised.

In cases of irreversible pulpitis, it is impossible to maintain the vitality of all pulpal tissues. At this stage of the inflammatory process, **vital extirpation** is the treatment of choice.

Histology

A The advanced dentin caries beneath the fissure has reached the pulpal tissues; note the accumulation of inflammatory cells. The root canal pulp exhibits several diffuse calcifications, but is inflammation-free.

B Within the coronal pulp, one notes a massive inflammatory cell infiltration with small areas of tissue disintegration.

C The bacteria within the dentinal tubules attract neutrophilic granulocytes. "Empty spaces" in the subodontoblastic layer represent micronecrosis, with pus accumulation and polymorphonuclear granulocytes.

D Granulocytes dominate both perivascularly as well as intravascularly; this is the picture of persisting chemotactic irritation. Larger "empty spaces" represent initial tissue necrosis. One also notes plasma cells and macrophages, which produce cytokines and chemokines, leading to chemoattraction of leukocytes. These mobilize monocytes, neutrophilic granulocytes, and other effector cells, attracting them to the focus of infection.

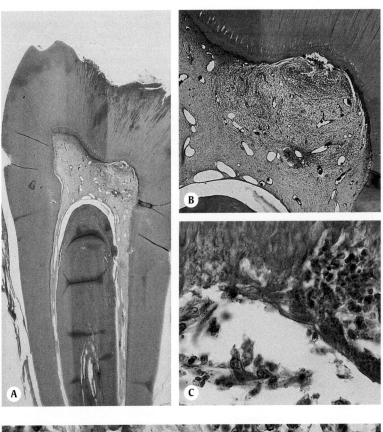

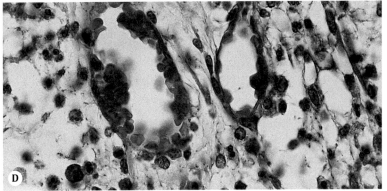

Bacterial Infection of the Pulpal Tissues

Of the ca. 600 bacterial species present in the oral cavity, only a small number are seen in an infected root canal. The frequency of individual bacteria can vary between 100 to over 10 million. The size of a periapical lesion correlates with the total number of bacteria and their species. A greater variety of bacterial species can be isolated from root canals in teeth with larger periapical lesions.

The dynamics of **bacterial infection** within root canals was studied in a series of animal experiments. In teeth whose pulpal tissues were infected with bacteria from the saliva and subsequently tightly sealed, early examinations revealed a preponderance of facultative anaerobes; after six months, however, the number of these bacteria had decreased to 2%. The proportion of obligate anaerobic bacterial strains increased with time. It was concluded that a selection mechanism within the root canal enhanced the development of specific environmental conditions.

Within root canals, bacteria often exist in **symbiosis**. For example, one often observes *Fusobacterium nucleatum* together with *Peptostreptococcus micros*, *Wolinella recta*, *Porphyromonas endodontalis*, and *Selenomonas sputigena*.

Numerous factors can influence bacterial colonization of the root canal. Some bacteria can use the metabolic by-products of other bacteria as nutrition. In addition, bacteriocin, which is released from certain microorganisms, can inhibit or enhance the growth of other bacteria.

Some bacteria in an infected root canal release enzymes that increase the pathogenicity of the bacteria. For example, immunoglobulins from the host organism can be inactivated by *P. asaccharolyticus* and *P. endodontalis*; *P. intermedia* and *P. gingivalis* degrade complement factor C3. Both are important opsonins for the phagocytosis of these bacteria during the host defense process. *P. gingivalis* can simultaneously break down proteinase inhibitors that are important for maintenance of the integrity of the still healthy tissues surrounding the infection.

A **necrotic pulp** without bacterial infection never leads to the formation of a periapical lesion. Only in the presence of bacteria will apical periodontitis develop.

A persisting microbial infection is the primary reason for endodontic failure. According to recently published studies, the microbial composition of a failed root canal procedure differ significantly from that of an untreated, infected canal: The necrotic pulp exhibits a **polymicrobial colonization**, consisting of four to seven species, predominantly anaerobes, in approximately equal numbers of gram-negative and gram-positive bacteria. In contrast, in previously treated root canals with persisting periapical lesions, usually only a single species (monoinfection) is found, usually *Enterococcus faecalis*. Gram-positive microorganisms predominate at 83.3%. In 57% one notes facultative anaerobes, and in 42.6% obligate anaerobic bacteria. The presence of *Peptostreptococcus* is usually associated with clinical symptoms.

Histology

A/B The progression of the carious process has led to exposure of the pulpal tissues, which exhibit tissue necrosis of the coronal pulp as well as large portions of the soft tissue within the root canals. Apical periodontitis is obvious in the periapical regions.

C Using histobacteriologic special stains, it is possible to identify the reddish-stained bacteria within the necrotic tissue.

D Coronal pulp and the coronal aspect of the root canal tissues contain bacterial conglomerates.

E This high power view reveals phagocytosed bacteria within neutrophilic granulocytes. This shows the active defense capability of the endodontium; however, once the bacterial infection becomes too massive, the host response is overwhelmed.

F Within the area of periapical inflammation, no bacteria can be identified histologically.

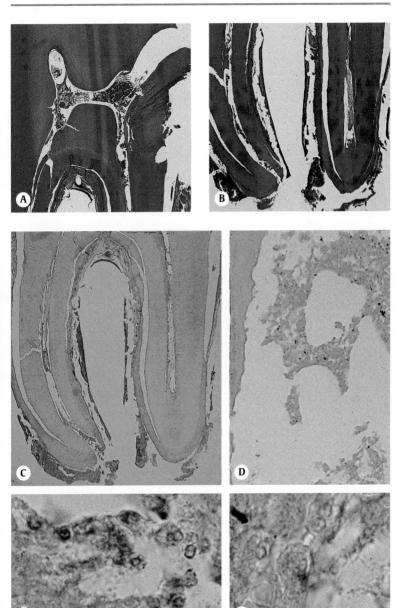

Pulpal necrosis is an irreversible condition characterized by tissue destruction. It can occur locally, or within the entire coronal pulp, or in both coronal and root canal pulp. The primary etiologic factor in pulpal necrosis is bacterial infection and the subsequent inflammatory host response; the expanse of the necrotic process is directly correlated with the magnitude of bacterial invasion.

Differences exist between coagulation necrosis and liquefaction necrosis. **Coagulation necrosis** involves lethal cell damage in which oxidative phosphorylation collapses as a result of damage to the mitochondria. Intracellular and transcellular transport processes shut down, and phospholipase-induced collapse of both cytoskeleton and cell membrane occurs. Released proteolysates attract granulocytes into the area of necrosis.

A special form of coagulation necrosis is **gangrene**. This represents a summary effect of necrosis with desiccation, which inhibits both bacterial growth and autolytic destruction ("dry type").

The "wet type" of necrosis is **liquefaction necrosis**, which is caused by a primary or secondary colonization by anaerobic bacteria. In liquefaction necrosis, enzymatic tissue destruction predominates.

If the carious process reaches the pulp and exposes it, studies demonstrate that there is always necrosis of the coronal pulpal tissues. The coronal pulp of all such teeth becomes partially or totally necrotic, but only in two-thirds of cases is the root canal pulp involved. Coronal pulp always exhibits bacteria, but in only one-third of teeth is the root canal colonized. In 90% of all patients studied, a periapical radiolucency occurs early on.

The condition of the pulpal tissues within the adjacent lateral canals corresponds to that of the suprajacent pulp. If the pulp of the primary canal is necrotic, the process extends also into the lateral canals; at such locations, a lateral lesion can also develop. If the pulp is vital, however, the lateral canals also maintain vital tissue.

In the case of **apical periodontitis**, the coronal pulp and some of the root canal pulp are already necrotically involved; however, there is usually remaining vital pulp tissue between the necrosis and the periapically inflamed tissues. As a result, with apical periodontitis the lateral canals are relatively seldom infected, and therefore the primary indication for apicoectomy with apical periodontitis is not fulfilled.

It is impossible to ascertain clinically the precise time point when bacterial infiltration of the pulpal tissue occurs. Long before carious exposure of pulpal tissue occurs, abscess formation and tissue necrosis begin. The etiology of early and severe pulpal destruction includes bacterial endotoxin, released by the death of gram-negative bacteria. High concentrations of endotoxin are inherently toxic and cause tissue necrosis; low doses, on the other hand, lead to elevated cell proliferation and collagen synthesis, as a manifestation of host response.

Bacteria elicit tissue necrosis, and are seldom observed outside the area of necrosis. Corresponding to the picture of a normal host response/reaction, the zones of necrosis are surrounded by neutrophilic granulocytes and macrophages that exhibit evidence of an active phagocytic process (bacteria contained within). Simultaneously, extracellularly released lysosomal products destroy the pulpal tissues. Bacteria penetrate not only into the necrotic area, but also into adjacent dentinal tubuli.

Appositions (fibrodenticles, diffuse dentin deposits), and also areas of **resorption**, occur in areas of necrosis.

Histology

A The carious process has led to coronal openings into the pulp chamber. The coronal pulp is necrotic and an abscess has formed.

B The tissue is lytically destroyed; no cell nuclei are stained.

C–E At the transition to the root canal pulp, one notes necrosis of the pulp tissues and in the apical direction an incipient tissue necrosis. In this region, one notes a massive accumulation of inflammatory cells. Coronally one sees a free denticle, which effectively closes the entrance to the root canal.

F–G Within the area of tissue destruction, one observes neutrophilic granulocytes, where enzyme release causes further tissue destruction.

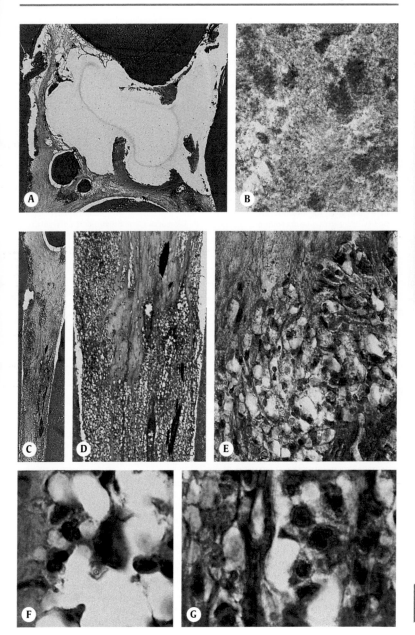

If the carious process progresses so far that the pulp chamber is actually opened clinically, pus can escape and the inflammatory reaction process will be quite different vis-à-vis closed pulpitis. Differentiation is made between chronic open **ulcerative** pulpitis and chronic open **hyperplastic** pulpitis. In contrast to closed pulpitis, these two forms of pulpitis are easily diagnosed clinically. As soon as the progression of caries leads to broad opening of the pulp chamber, any exudate can escape and this leads in most patients to a pain-free clinical situation.

With **chronic open ulcerative pulpitis**, there exist areas of tissue necrosis and ulceration as well as a large number of dead and necrotic cells. Adjacent to the necrotic foci, one observes lymphocytes, plasma cells, and macrophages, but the predominant superficial cell is the polymorphonuclear leukocyte. Beneath the now open dentin roof there exists an ulcerated pulpal surface.

Neutrophilic granulocytes and macrophages exhibit microorganisms both extracellularly and intracellularly. The vasculature exhibits a loosening of the endothelial cells, with subsequent transmigration of leukocytes.

With increased proliferation of the granulation tissue, this type of pulpitis becomes **chronic open hyperplastic pulpitis**. From the exposed pulp, granulation tissue begins to extrude, becoming a growing mass of tissue extruding from the usually wide coronal opening. The tissue is pink in color and globular in appearance; it may be colonized by cells from the marginal epithelium and subsequently become completely epithelialized. One differentiates between **"young pulp polyps,"** that consist of hyperplastic granulation tissue, and **"mature pulp polyps"** with their connective tissue and epithelialized surface. The multilayered squamous epithelium corresponds histologically and in terms of differentiation to the keratinized oral gingival epithelium.

The **differential diagnosis** must include pulp polyp, periodontal polyp (emanating from the cervical root surface), and fibrous gingival hyperplasia (emanating from the interdental gingiva).

Because of the bacterial infection of the pulpal tissue, open pulpitis must be treated by definitive removal of pulpal tissues up to the entrance of the root canals. Subsequently the canals are instrumented. Because in most patients complete tissue necrosis with initial periapical inflammation exists, the definitive root canal filling should be performed only after a one-month waiting period. Difficulties are most often associated only with the severe damage to the tooth crown and the consequences for subsequent restorative treatment of the endodontically treated tooth.

Histology

A The carious process has destroyed much of the dentin, and bacteria have entered the pulp chamber; the result is ulceration as well as a massive accumulation of inflammatory cells. From the ulcerative pulpal tissue, granulation tissue begins to emerge and literally grow out of the coronal opening. The bacterial infiltration of the coronal pulpal tissue leads to necrotization with tissue destruction; within the ulcerated tissue is an accumulation of polymorphonuclear leukocytes; at the transition to the root canals one observed a mononuclear leukocytic wall. Granulation tissue is also visible in the periapical area.

B The coronal pulpal tissue is epithelialized and consists primarily of dense connective tissue; it is collagen fiber-rich, relatively free of vasculature, and contains numerous nerve fibers that reach even to the epithelium, as well as areas of persisting chronic inflammatory infiltration.

C The surface is colonized by gingival epithelial cells and the multilayered squamous epithelium corresponds to that of a keratinized gingival epithelium.

D This enlarged view of the coronal third of the root canal reveals an infiltration with inflammatory cells, tissue components, as well as destruction of the odontoblastic layer.

E/F The inflammatory infiltrate is dominated by monocytes. In addition to lymphocytes, note also the plasma cells, an expression of a local immune reaction.

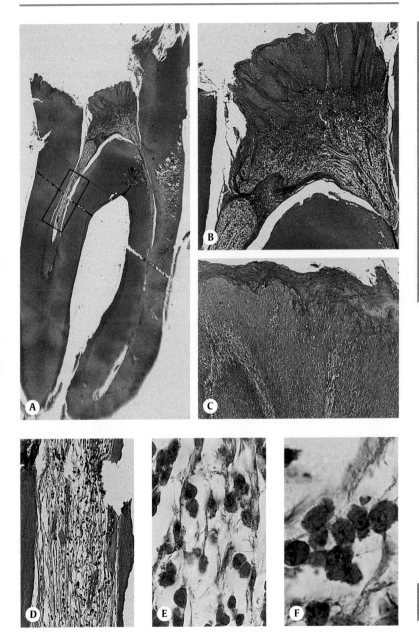

A mild hemorrhagic response occurs about four hours following experimental pulp exposure; within two days this response gives way to an intense cellular inflammatory infiltrate. A pulp polyp forms after seven days in 60% of patients; in 30%, necrosis occurs.

Studies employing vital microscopy demonstrate interruption of microcirculation 24 hours after cavity preparation. The severity of the inflammation directly correlates with the depth of the experimental cavity.

Pulp Capping with Calcium Hydroxide

Following exposure of the pulpal tissues and coverage with Ca(OH)$_2$ a three-layered necrosis ensues. The most superficial **zone of pressure necrosis** is followed by a **zone of liquefaction necrosis**, evoked by the chemical effect of hydroxyl ions. A distinct neutralization of the OH$^-$ ions occurs. Beneath these two layers, a **zone of coagulation necrosis** appears already one hour after pulp capping. As a result of this superficial necrosis, further hemorrhage is prevented, and a mild inflammation of the surrounding vital pulpal tissue is simultaneously elicited.

About 12 hours later, neutrophilic inflammatory cells migrate into the area, separated from the pulpal tissues by a fibrillar zone. After four days, proliferation of pulp cells occurs, and after seven days fibroblasts can be seen. These cells synthesize collagen at the boundary of the necrotic zone. Subsequently the collagen fibers mineralize, forming a layer of irregularly structured mineralized tissue.

Four weeks after pulp capping, one observes at the pulpal aspect a row of odontoblast-like cells, which probably derive from undifferentiated perivascular cells. Only three months later, a hard substance barrier forms from irregularly mineralized hard tissue; the barrier exhibits on the pulpal aspect tubuli-containing structures, and is bordered by odontoblasts.

Therefore, the **formation of hard substance** can be viewed as two phases: The first is a defense phase with cell death and inflammation. This **defense phase** is followed by a **repair phase** with the formation of a hard substance bridge. The alkalization caused by the calcium hydroxide is limited to the most superficial layers of pulpal tissue; a pH value drop can be measured immediately beneath the wound surface. As a result of vascular damage and expansion, bicarbonate is released. This buffer system protects the adjacent tissues.

The role of calcium hydroxide, particularly the calcium ions, has not been sufficiently clarified to date. It is known that the calcium forming the hard substance barrier derives exclusively from the adjacent pulpal tissues and not from the calcium hydroxide.

The formation of a hard substance bridge and healing of the pulpal wound can be negatively influenced by bacterial infection as well as by irritation caused by filling materials.

Histology

A Failure of direct pulp capping: The pulp was exposed, followed by a 10-second application of a low concentration acid, then the cavity was filled with glass ionomer cement. Thirty days later, the tooth was extracted.

B Opposite the cavity one observes necrotization of the pulpal tissues, and an adjacent inflammatory cell infiltrate.

C Section from the zone of necrosis: No hard tissue bridge has formed.

D The inflammatory cell infiltrate consists primarily of neutrophilic granulocytes surrounding the necrosis. No clinical symptoms of pain were reported.

E Formation of an incomplete hard substance bridge 90 days after pulp exposure and capping with glass ionomer cement.

F Following application of the capping material, further hemorrhage occurred between the pulpal tissue and the filling material. This explains the gap between the hard tissue formation and the filling material. A mild inflammation persists within the pulpal tissue.

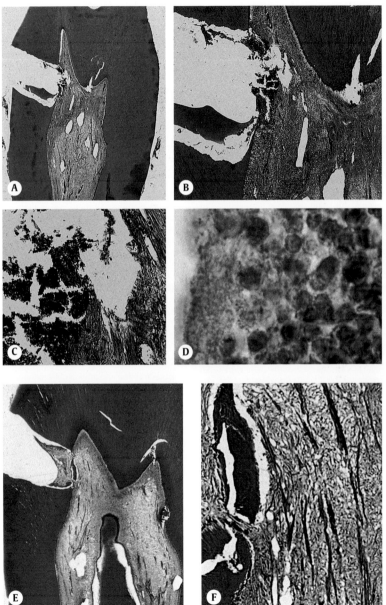

The ability of the pulp to form hard tissue is not limited only to the odontoblastic layer. **Fibrodentin depositions** are also observed in the form of denticles even in the center of the pulp. In our own histologic studies, we observed hard tissue deposits in both erupted and noneruptet primary and permanent teeth, and in both young and old persons.

Denticles, depending upon on their source, can be differentiated into **true** and **false** denticles, as well as with regard to their position vis-à-vis the canal wall into **adherent**, **free**, or **interstitial denticles**.

All regularly structured orthodenticles are anomalies of invagination, in which partial dentin protrusion occur within the pulp chamber. Complete dentin protrusions or projections can result in a **dens invaginatus.** Fibrodenticles must be differentiated from so-called true denticles with tubular dentin. The latter are rare, originating from breaks in the epithelial rests of the Hertwig sheath, around which odontoblasts are concentrically arranged.

Radially structured denticles exhibit a connection to the surrounding tissues via reticular fibers that surround the denticle and splay into it. On the other hand, lamella-shaped denticles exhibit only a loose connection to the individual dentin layers.

With regard to the origins of denticles and their classification, currently there exist various hypotheses. For example, an external influence may lead to cell death, around which a concentric denticle may form. In teeth with crown fractures, one observes mineralizations in 50% of patients, including both lamella-like denticles as well as diffuse deposits. In one-quarter of such cases, one observes inflammatory cells.

In addition, as a result of irreversible thermal irritation, there may be a circumscribed area of tissue or vascular disintegration, which leads to the formation of a layer of fibrodentin against the vital tissue as a sort of protective reaction. The origin of concentric, lamella-shaped denticles is likely pulpal vessels that are regularly found within the center of denticles. Such denticles are surrounded by pulpoblasts and reticular fibers.

Dissociation of odontoblasts out of the odontoblastic layer is unlikely. On the other hand, it seems possible that through secondary differentiation, new hard tissue-forming cells may derive from pulpal fibroblasts.

Diffuse mineralizations within the root canal, also called diffuse calcifications, are usually found along the vessels or along collagen fibers.

There is a significant increase in mineralizations in carious teeth compared with healthy teeth. In addition, as the carious process proceeds there is an increase in the number and expanse of denticles. Additional causes for the existence of denticles include severe abrasion and erosion, twisting of the vascular system, e.g., as a result of surgical procedures, and occlusal parafunctions as well as traumatic influences upon the tooth.

Expansive mineralizations within the root canal can make canal instrumentation more difficult.

Histological investigations have shown that the occurrence of denticles must not necessarily have any connection with pulpal problems. For example, in 57 teeth with such calcifications, not one patient reported pain symptoms. Even hard tissue formations in old teeth, even up to almost complete obliteration of the root canal, can be completely free of clinical symptoms.

Histology

A Fibrodenticle in the process of increasing adherence to the root canal wall by means of active secondary dentin formation.

B Denticle attachment to the canal wall in secondary dentin (the cleft is an artifact).

C Onion skin-shaped, irregularly formed fibrodenticle.

D Free fibrodentin denticle with hard tissue-forming pulpoblasts at the periphery, and tissue inclusions within.

E Rudiments of vessels in the center of a denticle.

F Attachment of flat, hard tissue-forming cells at the periphery of the denticle. These connective tissue cells are often referred to as "pulpoblasts."

G Enlarged section from the center of the denticle, showing vessels and rudiments of cells.

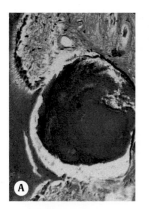

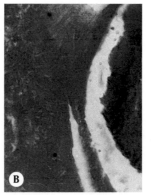

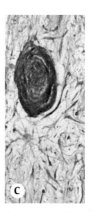

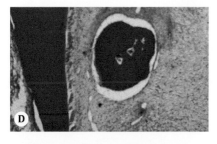

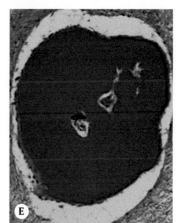

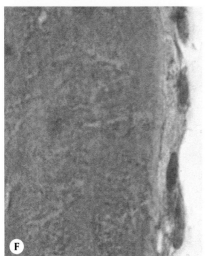

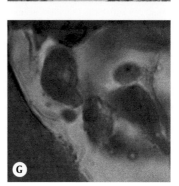

Resorptive processes in the dentition may affect enamel, dentin, and cementum. Depending upon whether the resorptions initiate within the pulp or within the periodontium, one can differentiate between **internal** and **external resorption**.

Whether they occur on vital or nonvital teeth, root resorption is the result of dentoclastic activity. The causes of internal resorption include chronic inflammation through tissue necrosis within the pulp, resulting in loss of function and loss of odontoblasts. Even mechanical trauma can lead to internal resorption in 2% of patients. There still remains today much speculation concerning explanation for the etiology of internal resorption.

Inflammatory stimuli that could elicit or enhance internal resorption include three possibilities:
- cytokines such as IL-1 and TNF
- prostaglandin PGE_2
- possibly increased internal tissue pressures. However, several case reports demonstrate that even on healthy, not-yet-erupted teeth internal resorption may be in evidence.

As is the case with progression of caries (and also periodontitis!), internal resorption appears to be characterized by phases of active resorption alternating with phases of remission; during the latter, new hard tissue can be laid down in the form of secondary dentin.

The **internal granuloma** is a very rare occurrence; maximum 1.6% of all individuals are affected. If it is localized to the coronal pulp chamber, a variably large reddish enamel spot may be in evidence (**pink spot disease**). In most patients, tooth sensitivity test remains positive. Differentiation of an internal granuloma from an **external granuloma** can only be achieved with several radiographs taken using various excentric ray projections. If the radiolucency does not change in localization, then the lesion is clearly an internal resorption.

Only if the resorption perforates and permits contact with the oral cavity (also possible via deep periodontal pockets) will bacteria invade the pulpal tissues, and this can result in necrosis as well as the formation of a periapical lesion. If there is lateral perforation without an opening to the oral cavity, the pulp will remain vital.

In a very comprehensive study, Heithersay examined the potential predisposing factors for invasive cervical resorption. Orthodontic treatment was the most frequent single factor, occurring in 21.2% of all patients and 24.1% of all teeth. Trauma was the second most frequent (15.1%), and bleaching (3.9%) was the third most important single factor. In 21% of patients, combinations of the individual factors were involved.

If an internal resorption is diagnosed, and if there is no perforation, **pulpectomy** is the treatment of choice. In such cases, it is prudent to perform thorough and lengthy rinsing of the root canal with 5% sodium hypochlorite solution to assure removal of all tissue debris, because the entire root canal often cannot be completely instrumented mechanically. Root canal filling is performed using the vertical condensation technique. In cases of resorptions that have perforated, it is usually necessary to employ a combined endodontic–surgical procedure.

Histology

A Porcine anterior tooth following preparation of a cavity and filling with silicate cement.

B The enlarged section of an internal resorption exhibits a high number of vessels. Giant cells are visible at the periphery.

C Visible are neutrophilic granulocytes and lymphocytes as well as multinucleated giant cells.

D Adjacent to the tubular dentin one sees multinucleated giant cells (dentinoclasts), which have created resorption lacunae (Howship lacunae).

E Individual dentinoclasts as multinucleated giant cells exhibiting clear polarity. The dentin surface exhibits a ruffled border. The cellular processes may exhibit ameboid mobility; lysosomal enzymes destroy dentin matrix. The remaining organic matrix is phagocytozed.

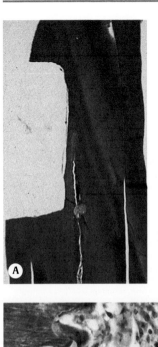

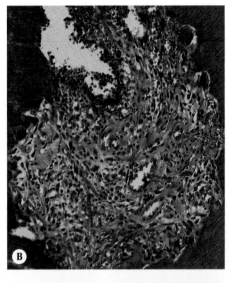

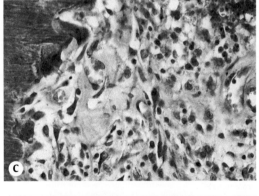

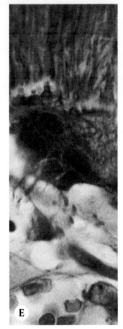

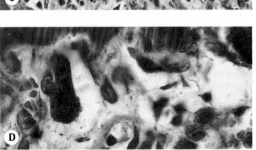

A periapical lesion will occur only in the presence of **bacteria in the root canal**. This was demonstrated as early as 1965 by Kakehashi and coworkers using germ-free rats; the teeth developed periapical inflammation only after bacterial inoculation. If the teeth were only trephined and then left open to the germ-free oral milieu, no apical periodontitis developed. Similar results were reported in monkey experiments. Following necrotization of the pulpal tissues, no periapical lesions developed if the trephination opening was completely closed to the oral cavity.

In periapical lesions, bacteria are always detectable within the root canal, distributed as well as attaching to the dentin walls, and within the dentinal tubules. In 18% of teeth exhibiting apical periodontitis, bacteria were found in the periapical tissues, in some cases *Actinomycosis*.

Acute apical periodontitis is characterized histopathologically as an exudate of polymorphonuclear granulocytes and macrophages, limited to the osteoclastically widened periodontal ligament space. Macrophages play the dominant role in the degradation of immune complexes and complement complexes, while neutrophilic granulocytes provide defense against foreign body substances. Macrophages attract bacterial antigens and elevate their immunogenicity. This leads to a further massive accumulation of neutrophilic granulocytes with attendant tissue necrosis, disintegration, and abscess formation.

In **periapical abscesses**, the necrotic tissue around the root apex is filled with bacteria and is demarcated by a wall of neutrophilic granulocytes.

The flora of a periapical abscess is polymicrobial, but with participation of only a few bacterial species; gram-negative anaerobic rods and peptostreptococci predominate. Periapical abscesses contain black-pigmenting bacterial species, which are believed to play an important role in the etiology of periapical lesions. In 63% of lesions, *P.intermedia* is found, and *P.endodontalis* in 53% of patients of with apical periodontitis.

Acute apical periodontitis is a **very painful condition**, without clear radiographic **periapical radiolucency**. Edema fluid and neutrophilic granulocytes fill the periapical space between tooth and bone. This leads to irritation of the nerve endings, a condition that is further aggravated by external forces upon the tooth. The tooth reacts with exquisite pain upon percussion. The patient feels that the tooth is elongated and may report premature occlusal contact.

With a primary acute lesion, the radiograph will not exhibit any significant radiolucency. With the influx primarily of neutrophilic granulocytes into the periodontal ligament space, enzymes are subsequently released, which activate osteoclasts; these lead eventually to bone resorption. In most cases, there is also histologic evidence of proliferation of epithelial rest cells of Malassez, which can later lead to cyst formation.

An acute apical periodontitis does not require complete necrosis of the entire pulp. Even with partial necrosis, endotoxins may play a role as etiologic factors for acute apical reactions.

Histology

A The apical region of the root canal pulp is infiltrated by inflammatory cells; the toxins that are released during the inflammatory process elicit the periapical inflammatory reaction.

B Coronally one observes necrotic tissue, but further apically the tissue contains only individual inflammatory cells. The cavitations and apparent dissolution of the pulpal tissues from the canal wall are artifacts.

C Enlarged section from the coronal zone of necrosis exhibiting a wall of neutrophilic granulocytes.

D Periapical accumulation of inflammatory cells; also the simultaneous appearance of resorption lacunae indicate dentinoclastic and osteoclastic activity.

E The enlarged section from the periapical region exhibits a massive accumulation of acute polymorphonuclear granulocytes.

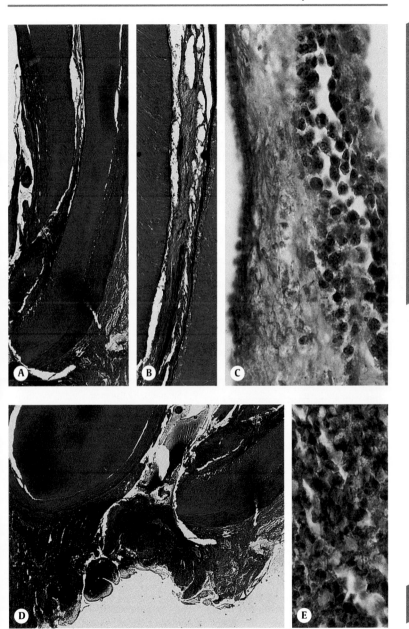

Following experimental induction of apical periodontitis in rat molars, histologic examination revealed an **active phase** with aggressive bone destruction between seven and 20 days, and subsequently a **chronic phase** with less expansion. Morphometric analysis showed that lymphocytes dominated after 15 days, but also up to 90 days (50–60% of all cells), followed by polymorphonuclear leukocytes (25–40%), macrophages and monocytes, plasma cells, and fibroblasts. Helper T cells dominated in the acute lesions while suppressor T cells dominated in chronic periapical lesions.

T helper cells play an important role in bone resorption, while **T suppressor cells** stabilize the periapical lesion in the sense of rendering it chronic. T helper cells induce: (1) the production of an interferon that stimulates macrophages to secrete the bone resorption factor IL-1; (2) the production of a bone-resorption cytokine; and (3) T-helper-cell factors for antibody production and the formation of immune complexes. High concentrations of IL-1 also inhibit new bone formation by suppressing protein synthesis by osteoblasts.

Chronic apical periodontitis is **clinically asymptomatic**. There is a direct relationship between the size of the periapical lesion and the concentration or expansion of the bacterial infiltration and tissue necrosis within the root canal.

The chronic periapical lesion consists of three to four primary components:

- a focus of infiltrate consisting of lymphocytes and plasma cells
- centrally or at the borders, granulation tissue with fibroblasts may exist, or may be completely absent
- epithelial rest cells of Malassez may proliferate (cyst formation!)
- one observes a connective tissue capsule with fibroblasts and collagen fiber bundles.

The elevated antibody concentration in acute lesions and the reduction of antibodies following endodontic therapy demonstrate that the instrumentation of the root canal and the removal of bacterially infected tissues in chronic apical periodontitis is the **treatment** of choice.

In summary, chronic apical periodontitis is a clinically asymptomatic inflammation where-in a balance between bacterial infection and host response exists in a state of "stand off."

The frequently used term **granuloma** is inappropriate for this condition and leads to confusion because the lesion of chronic apical periodontitis does not present the classical monocytic/macrophage-dominated lesion, but rather an inflammation characterized by lymphocytes and plasma cells. In addition, depending upon the degree of activity, polymorphonuclear cells may also be present.

Teeth with small periapical lesions generally react positively to a sensitivity test, but with larger periapical lesions one does not observe any reaction to an electric or thermal vitality test.

Histology

A The chronic periapical lesion is surrounded by a firm connective capsule that contains mast cells, fibroblasts, and collagen fiber bundles. In the center, one notes a focus of infiltrate consisting primarily of mononuclear inflammatory cells such as lymphocytes, plasma cells, and macrophages.

B One notes strands of epithelium immediately adjacent to the apex as well as distributed in bizarre formations within the central zone of the periapical lesion. These strands of epithelium probably derive from epithelial rest cells (Malassez), but the latter are found in only 20–40% of all chronic apical periodontitis lesions.

C Within the granulation tissue are fibroblasts and mononuclear inflammatory cells, and in the center of the lesion one also notes encapsulated microabscesses.

D This enlarged section reveals stands of epithelium and a mononuclear infiltration; note also the encapsulated microabscesses that could provide the initial substrate for a prospective cyst epithelium.

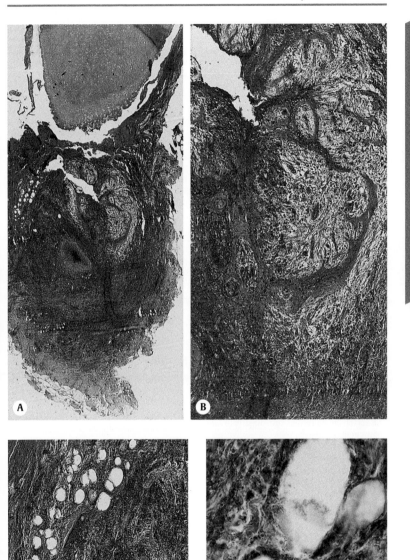

Various authors have reported the incidence of radicular cysts to be between 6–55%; however, based on serial sections, it is only between 15–17%. In a clinical and histologic study of 230 root-tip biopsies with radiographic periapical radiolucencies and clinical symptoms, only 14 cysts (6%) could be demonstrated.

In a radiograph, chronic apical periodontitis appears as a round to oval, usually sharply demarcated radiolucency. Only seldom is a diffuse border observed. In the radiograph, average size radicular cysts cannot be differentiated from the lesion of chronic apical periodontitis; however, beyond a 10-mm diameter and with increasing size, the percentage of cysts increases. Even with radiolucencies of 10–15 mm, at least 50% proved **not** to be cysts. Only the use of computerized tomographic examination can permit a clear differential diagnosis.

The **radicular cyst** is defined as an area of chronic inflammation exhibiting a closed central cavity surrounded by an epithelial lining.

The cyst develops–in three stages–from a pre-existing chronic apical periodontitis:
- in the phase of **initiation,** dormant Malassez rest cells begin to proliferate
- during phase 2, a central cavity lined by epithelium develops
- during the **growth phase**, the cyst enlarges in size as a result of osmotic and other factors that stimulate bone resorption.

The established radicular cyst consists of four components:
- the connective tissue capsule
- a subepithelial zone of chronic inflammatory infiltrate
- the epithelial cyst wall
- the cystic lumen.

In addition to desquamative, necrotic epithelial cells and cholesterol, the cystic lumen also contains inflammatory cells and debris from the resorbed osseous tissue. The epithelial cystic wall is a multilayered squamous epithelium infiltrated by granulocytes, macrophages, and lymphocytes. The subepithelial zone contains T and B lymphocytes as well as plasma cells.

Most recently, a differentiation has been drawn between **true cysts** with their completely epithelial lined central cavity and **pocket cysts** whose central lumen is open to the root canal. Of 256 periapical lesions, 9% were classified as true cysts and 6% as periapical pocket cysts.

The existence of two classes of radicular cysts, as well as the impossibility to differentiate radiographically or clinically between cysts and apical periodontitis, brings with it important therapeutic consequences.

The **treatment for periapical lesions** involves the removal of the cause of the inflammatory reaction, the instrumentation of the root canal as well as a closure that prevents bacterial invasion. Because the radiograph cannot provide a definitive differential diagnosis and the fact that the histologic picture is unknown, the first treatment for any periapical lesion is exclusively **conventional** therapy.

Periapical pocket cysts usually heal completely. However, it is unlikely that true cysts can be successfully treated conventionally.

Histology

A Within the lumen of the radicular cyst, one observes cholesterol crystals surrounded by the epithelial cystic wall.

B The epithelial wall is a multilayered squamous epithelium.

C Within the cystic cavity, one notes cholesterol crystals, necrotic tissue, neutrophilic granulocytes, and mononuclear leukocytes.

D The remnants of lamellar bone within the cystic cavity indicate the resorptive capacity of the cystic tissues.

E Multinuclear giant cells are both an indication of a possible foreign body reaction as well as of osteoclastic activity; adjacent plasma cells produce antibodies, primarily IgG and IgA, and lesser amounts of IgM and IgE; this is an expression of an immune reaction.

F Lymphocytes are primarily T cells, less often B cells, in a ratio of 3:1.

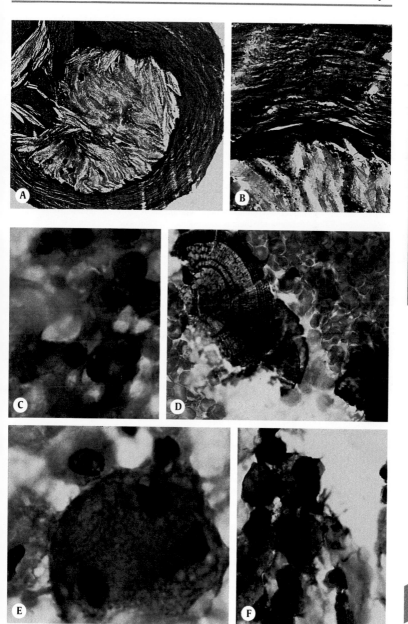

Elimination of pain, and the **cause** of that pain, is a primary goal in dentistry. A precise diagnosis and the subsequent treatment plan result from thorough consideration of subjective and objective clinical and radiographic criteria.

Symptoms described by the patient lead in most cases to a definitive diagnosis. After collecting the medical and dental history, the next step is a comprehensive extraoral and intraoral examination. Due to their anatomical peculiarities, however, diseases of the pulp and the periapical periodontal tissue cannot be directly inspected.

In addition to objective clinical findings, the subjective phenomenon of **pain** provides a most important criterion for ascertainment of the condition of the pulp; however, there is no general relationship between the histologic condition of the pulp and the individual clinical symptoms, especially pain. Pain elicited by cold indicates a reversible inflammatory process in the pulp; pain elicited by heat as well as persistent attacks of pain, especially at night, indicate an irreversible pulpitis.

If a patient presents with pain, it is important to clarify the etiology of that pain, i.e., is it of dentogenic origin or does it derive from neighboring oral structures. Clarification must involve comprehensive examination of the marginal periodontal tissues, including pocket depth measurements.

Examination of the patient includes medical and dental history, **extraoral** and **intraoral findings**, as well as establishing possible differential diagnoses. The patient's own subjective descriptions will provide hints concerning his/her dental as well as medical problems.

There is no medical contraindication for performing endodontic treatment. Nevertheless, any medical conditions as well as the psychic frame of mind of the patient should be taken into consideration. The **medical history** must include all medical conditions or medications being taken that might in any way influence endodontic treatment or which might be in any way influenced the dental treatment itself.

Systemic diseases such as rheumatic fever, coronary heart diseases, hypertension, as well as diabetes must be determined during collection of the medical history. The danger of bacterially induced endocarditis must be evaluated and such patients appropriated covered with antibiotics.

The **dental history** includes data that are important for treatment planning. During data collection, a summary of the patient's history of pain must be documented. The development of the present pain circumstance should be recorded using the patient's own words. The patient's previous visits to the dentist should be recorded. The pain history must include considerations of the type, time frame of occurrence, elicitation situations, and the site of the pain, as well as pain radiation to circumscribed regions. Questions concerning bleeding or pus release from the gingiva, food impaction between teeth and elevated tooth mobility may be significant.

Case Report

A In a 25-year-old female, a painless, ulcerated, erythematous lesion of 1 cm diameter was noted on the chin; it had persisted for more than one year.

B The radiograph clearly revealed a sharply demarcated radiolucency in the periapical region.

C Swelling of the left side of the face, without any attendant dental pain.

D The radiograph revealed a large periapical lesion around the root apices of the maxillary first molar, which included the palatal root.

E Extraoral fistula exhibited pus release on the right side of the mandible. The differential diagnosis should include an ulcer because considerable tissue loss has occurred; another possibility, an aphthous ulcer, or even carcinoma (rare).

F After removal of the old restoration from tooth 46, an old pulp exposure was visible; the carious dentin had been treated by the dentist with a direct pulp cap procedure.

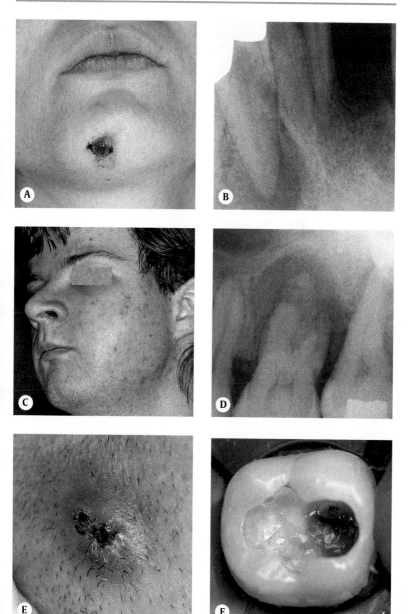

The **extraoral examination** involves consideration of normal findings as well as pathological changes, and it is enhanced by the patient's own statements.

External facial form and features are recorded as symmetrical or exhibiting asymmetric defects. The facial skin may exhibit abnormalities such as fistulae, erythema, or pallor, which may necessitate further clarification because they may indicate possible intraoral pathology.

The **neurologic examination** includes testing of motor function, sensitivity, and movement function. A bilateral comparison of the sensation of external stimuli is used to test the patient's ability to differentiate between a blunt and a sharp stimulus.

Examination of the **lymph nodes** in the face and jaw region can provide clues about inflammatory, infectious, or tumor-like disorders. Palpation is performed bimanually and with comparison left to right; painful lymph nodes are an indication of an acute inflammation.

The visual **intraoral examination** consists of a search for swelling, erythema, fistula, suppuration, dental caries, tooth discoloration and mobility, dental restorations, and a comprehensive evaluation of the periodontal supportive apparatus and the entire dentition.

Some or all of these examination procedures should be employed: palpation, percussion, determination of tooth mobility, periodontal examination, functional occlusal analysis, infraction test, sensitivity/vitality test, transillumination, selective anesthesia test, and radiographic examinations.

The **percussion** of an affected tooth may provide a sure sign, even in the earliest pathological involvement. The question is whether a periodontal or an endodontic etiology is present, or an occlusal trauma in combination with marginal periodontitis. The percussion test should also be performed on adjacent teeth in order to ascertain clear differences in the intensity of elicited pain.

Palpation in the vestibular fold near the **apical** region of the root tips will provide clues concerning pressure sensitivity and infiltration as well as the presence of swelling and even fluctuation. Applying pressure to the vestibular tissue can aid in the diagnosis of a fistula because pressure may elicit efflux of exudate.

In addition to the radiograph, transillumination may expose caries, tooth fracture, or other pathologic conditions. The use of targeted anesthesia may make it possible to detect the affected tooth. The percussion test may also provide additional important diagnostic clues; especially vertical or horizontal percussion sensitivity provides differential diagnostic conclusions. Having the patient bite upon a wooden tongue blade can provide evidence concerning tooth fracture or infraction during loading or unloading of the occlusion.

Before initiating endodontic treatment it is important to examine all of the remaining dentition. Does the affected tooth have an antagonist that justifies maintaining the affected tooth, and is prosthetic reconstruction even possible? Endodontic treatment is indicated only if maintenance of the tooth is necessary for prosthetic or other functional reasons.

Case Presentation

A Discolored restorations should be carefully checked for marginal imperfections.

B The maxillary incisor exhibits deep and penetrating caries; plaque accumulation within the cingulum was the point of initiation for the carious destruction.

C The buccal perforation was elicited by corrosion of the build-up post.

D In addition to discoloration of the tooth crown, note the swelling and the fistula, indicating periapical inflammation.

E Discoloration of the maxillary central incisor; a radiograph revealed root canal filling material extending into the coronal pulp chamber.

F Penetration of Toxavit through the inadequate temporary restoration, with periodontal tissue damage and persisting pain.

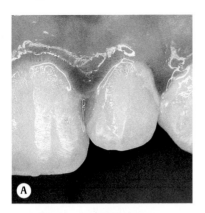

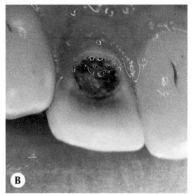

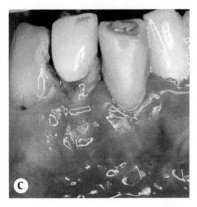

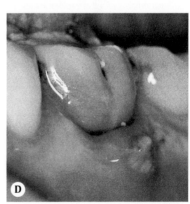

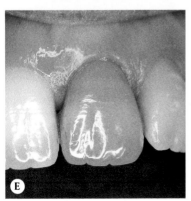

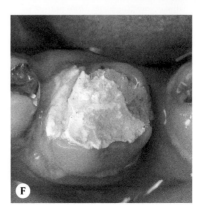

The endodontic sensitivity test is frequently, if incorrectly, referred to as a **vitality** test, even though it does not provide specific information regarding the histopathologic condition of the pulpal tissue. Nevertheless, it is a helpful test for differentiation of pulpal diseases.

Cold Test and Electric Sensitivity Test

Electrical or thermal sensitivity tests provide clues as to whether the pulpal tissue has been severely damaged or not. **Cold tests** are the most predictive. Any exact differentiations between clinically healthy pulp, reversible pulpitis, or irreversible pulpitis is, however, usually not possible using this test alone, because intact nerve tissue generally persists even in areas with severe inflammation and tissue necrosis. Even when periapical radiolucencies are noted, the sensitivity test may still be positive.

The cold test using dry ice has significant advantages over other sensitivity tests. Because an isolating moisture layer is formed beneath the CO_2 ice at temperatures above 0˚C, this test procedure is not damaging to the tooth or its surrounding tissue. Only after contact for two minutes or more will enamel be compromised.

Electric sensitivity test procedures are based upon the special conductivity of tooth hard structure. Within the device, the electrical impulse is established according to the impedance of the tooth, so that if the test probe inadvertently slides onto the oral mucosa the current is broken; thus, a false-positive result is prevented.

The electrode, usually made of conductive rubber, is placed onto the dried tooth surface. The electrical circuit is closed via the handpiece, and via a metal mouth mirror in the clinician's hand.

Young teeth with wide-open apical foramina have not yet fully developed their sensitivity, thus false-negative responses can occur. In addition, following trauma, the sensitivity test may prove negative for days or even weeks.

The electrical sensitivity test cannot be used on teeth with metal crowns, or on ceramic crowns because of the isolator effect.

False-negative responses may occur in teeth with expansive and advanced caries. The electrical test is **contraindicated** in patients with a cardiac pacemaker.

Heat Test

The heat test is indicated for the diagnosis of advanced pulpitis, but is only a confirmatory test.

Clinical Examination

A A temperature of 26–30˚C is achieved after four seconds of cold application. This elicits a pain reaction. Within the pulp, the temperature actually drops only about 0.2˚C. Ice cubes drop the temperature to –20˚C; cryogenic sprays, applied to the tooth surface on a cotton pellet, drop the temperature to –40˚C. Compressed dry ice may achieve even –70˚C.

B The electrical sensitivity test is simple and reliable. The tooth surface must be dry. The end of the pulp tester probe must be moistened, e.g., with toothpaste. Using the device with rubber gloves can lead to false readings because of the insulation. Simplest is to permit the electrical circuit to close when the metal portion of an instrument handle contacts the clinician's hand.

C Extraoral bimanual palpation of the lymph nodes.

D The buccal surface of the root is palpated in the vestibule, and the patient is asked about any sensitivity.

E Palpation of the palate follows the course of the root surfaces and adjacent tissues.

F Percussion sensitivity of a tooth is a sign of the presence of periapical inflammation. Root fractures can also be detected by percussion or by the biting test. The vital percussion test should also always be performed on the adjacent teeth for comparative purposes.

G Horizontal percussion using a mirror handle.

H Biting test on a wooden tongue blade. Pain upon release of biting force indicates an infraction, a vertical or horizontal tooth fracture.

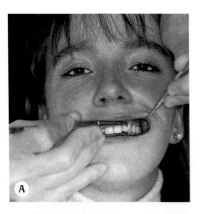
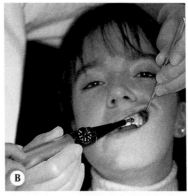

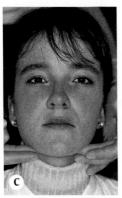
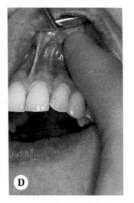
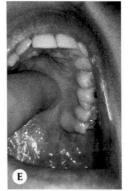

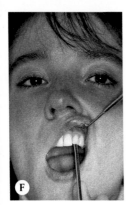
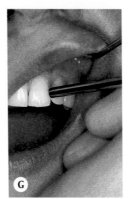
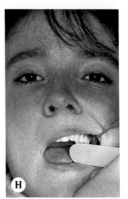

In addition to the clinical findings, radiographs have special significance for the determination of therapy. For example, in the posterior segments, 30–70% more dental caries will be diagnosed compared with clinical examination alone. It is astounding to note the differences in diagnosis by different examiners of the same radiograph: Interexaminer agreement is often less than 50%. When the same films were examined eight months later, only 88% of examiners agreed with their initial diagnosis!

Roentgen rays emanate in a rectilinear mode. An enlargement of the object is therefore unavoidable. Nevertheless, such enlargement is smaller if the distance between focus and tooth is greater and if the distance between the tooth and the radiographic film is smaller. A uniform enlargement results if the plane of the tooth and the plane of the film are parallel and the central ray is directed perpendicularly. This is precisely the situation when the **right angle technique** is employed. Using this method, the radiographic film is affixed in a holding device that is attached to the tube, and thus the central ray is oriented perpendicular to the middle of the film. In order to compensate for the object enlargement and any geometric blur, a long cone is required (large tooth-focus distance). The right angle technique permits reproducible radiographs.

Using the **bisecting angle technique**, the central ray projects perpendicularly upon the bisected plane between the tooth and the film. This technique is always associated with a certain irregular enlargement of some segments of the jaw. The advantage of the bisecting angle technique is that there is no necessity for a film holder device, or for a long cone.

In endodontics, an apical projection is preferred in the vertical aspect. In the horizontal direction, the central ray should course orthoradially, e.g., it impacts perpendicularly upon the tooth tangent and the radiographic film. Because any radiograph can only provide a two-dimensional view of a three-dimensional object, it is often prudent to also take radiographs from excentric angles. For such films, the central ray impacts more from either the distal or the mesial of the dental tangent. These are referred to as **mesial or distal excentric radiographs**. These radiographs often

make it possible to diagnosis additional root canals that were masked on the standard orthoradial projection.

In the radiograph, pathologic alterations will appear as **radiolucency** in cases of hard tissue destruction, or as **radiopacity** in cases of hard tissue accumulation. A periapical lesion in cases of chronic apical periodontitis manifests as a radiolucency due to bone resorption around the root tip. With a typical mineral content of 52% in cortical bone, a loss of 6.6% of osseous mineral is sufficient to render a periapical lesion radiographically visible. Thus, lesions of trabecular bone can be differentiated from the cortical element. Only the removal of the transition zone between trabecular and cortical bone, which cannot be anatomically differentiated on a radiograph, can lead to radiographically visible alterations because of the differences in consistency of the two osseous structures.

Case Presentation

A Mandibular molar in an orthoradial roentgen ray projection.

B Occlusal clinical view; the distal canal entrance is not clearly visible.

C This radiograph was taken with a slight distal excentric projection; visible are two "root shadows," which lead to the conclusion of two separate distal root canals.

D Following instrumentation of three root canals and coronal expansion to size 110, an additional canal entrance is noted distally.

E In the final radiograph, only three canals have obviously been instrumented and filled. Over the long term, this is a program for failure.

F Schematic depiction of the orthoradial (1) as well as the mesial excentric (3) and the distal excentric (2) projections. With the orthoradial projection, the central ray projects perpendicularly upon the expected tooth tangent, while the excentric projections from mesial or distal are divergent from the orthoradial.

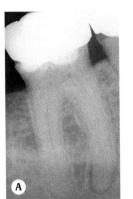

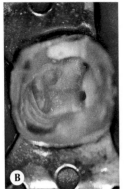

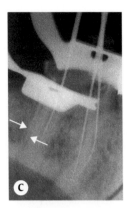

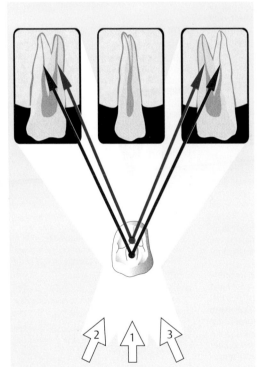

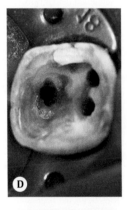

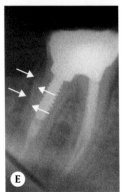

Emergency Treatment

Pain of endodontic origin is the most frequent complaint by patients in any dental practice. Carious lesions, including also secondary caries, are the primary etiology (88%), followed by cusp fractures, cervical hypersensitivity, and traumatic occlusion. Pain of endodontic origin often leads to organizational problems in the practice because these patients must be helped as quickly as possible until they are pain-free. If this goal is not achieved, the patient is often dissatisfied with the dentist's professional capability! One of the most frequent reasons for seeking a new dentist is the inability to deal quickly and effectively with pain of endodontic origin.

Treatment for dental pain must be preceded by a **definitive diagnosis**, which must differentiate between reversible or irreversible pulpitis, necrosis, or other apical pathology. Dental pain may be elicited by heat, cold, or sweet or sour foods and drinks. The pain may be very intense, but the pain usually is of short duration.

Reversible pulpitis is characterized by a narrow corridor of symptoms; the transition into irreversible pulpitis is indistinct, and definitive diagnosis is often very difficult. With reversible pulpitis, the carious process has not yet opened into the pulp; in some patients there may also be a fractured restoration or exposed dentin.

The situation may involve a positive sensitivity test as well as a negative percussion test, and the radiograph will usually depict deep caries or an old restoration with secondary caries. The radiograph usually does not reveal periapical pathology.

The dentist's reaction to the definitive diagnosis must be to pursue a goal of maintaining the tooth's vitality while simultaneously eliminating the patient's pain.

The initial **therapeutic** measure is therefore to completely remove all old restorations and all carious dentin; in **no case** must residual caries be allowed to remain *in situ*. Only these measures can ensure that no additional irritation of the pulpal tissue will occur.

To prevent the recurrence of clinical pain symptoms, extremely careful clinical procedures are indicated. The cavity must be covered using a zinc oxide-eugenol (ZnOE) dressing, with a low eugenol content and without

additives; a manually mixed glass ionomer cement with low fluid content may also be employed. A composite restoration with "total bonding" is contraindicated, likewise dentin bonding or phosphate cements.

Only after a minimum of 48 hours without pain symptoms can a **definitive restoration** with a biologically neutral cement base and definitive coverage be placed.

Direct pulp capping or even vital amputation is contraindicated in patients with pain; this approach, when employed for whatever reason, is only a temporary measure.

If pain persists or becomes more severe, these are symptoms of an **irreversible pulpitis**. In such cases, complete root canal debridement and subsequent filling must be performed.

Case Presentation

A This patient experienced pain in the maxillary anterior segment since placement of the composite restorations four months previously. The restorations could be easily lifted out with an explorer, revealing obvious caries that had not been completely removed. Subsequently, the caries was completely excavated and the cavities were covered with a zinc oxide-eugenol temporary restoration.

B The teeth were not percussion sensitive. The radiograph depicts a slight widening of the periodontal ligament space on the lateral incisor.

C Already the next morning, the patient presented in the office with an obvious swelling in the right infraorbital region; this was a clear indication that the initial diagnosis of reversible pulpitis was incorrect. It was therefore impossible to maintain the vitality of the involved teeth.

D It was necessary to make an incision, and pus release was achieved. On the following days the patient was free of symptoms.

E Two days later, all three root canals were debrided and a calcium hydroxide dressing was placed in the canals.

F Three weeks later, the patient was symptom-free and the definitive root canal fillings were performed.

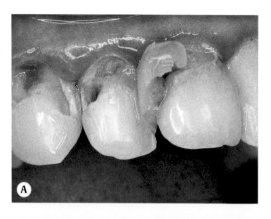

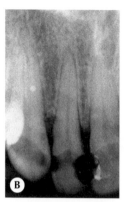

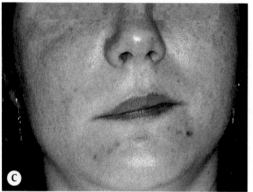

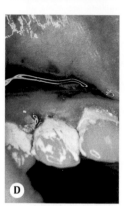

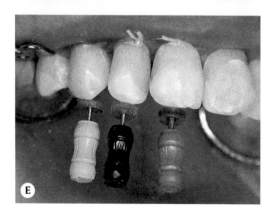

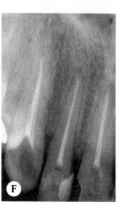

According to the International Association for the Study of Pain (IASP), pain is defined as an unpleasant sensation and a disturbing sensation that is attended by actual or potential tissue damage. **Acute pain** is always associated with some sudden or acute circumstance. On the other hand, according to established definitions, **chronic pain** is uninterrupted pain of three to six months' duration, which negatively influences cognitive/emotional status through disturbance of personal awareness, mood, or social behavior, as well as physiologic-organic status through inhibition of function. The differentiation between chronic and/or acute pain is a convenient clinical differentiation, but it is really based upon vague temporal criteria. A true and objective differentiation between acute and chronic pain in actual dental practice is difficult to define.

The transition from acute to chronic pain is characterized physiologically by the release of prostaglandins and neuropeptides, a reduction of the level of excitability, an elevation of neuronal discharge, and the development of spontaneous neuron activity. Dormant nociceptive afferent nerve fibers are recruited. It is also possible that a sensitization of central neurons with expansion of the receptive fields and loss of inhibitory mechanisms occurs.

The dental pulp is enervated afferently by thinly myelinized A_δ fibers and unmyelinized C fibers; both are responsible for the transmission of pain sensation. The former provide for a discrete and sharp pain, while the latter elicit a diffuse and poorly localizable pain sensation. The afferent C fibers appear primarily to be activated by temperatures above 43°C, while A_δ fibers react mainly to mechanical and osmotic stimuli.

Three theories for the existence of dentin pain remain under discussion: (1) the hydrodynamic theory with the movement of fluid within the dentinal tubuli; (2) the direct nerve stimulation theory; as well as (3) odontoblasts with receptor function and synaptic transmission.

The **hydrodynamic theory** assumes a fluid flow within the dentinal tubuli, influenced or initiated by chemical, osmotic or physical stimuli. Subsequently this movement is transmitted to the odontoblastic processes and this leads to stimulation of free nerve endings (not yet definitively identified).

The theory is that sensitive nerve endings are stimulated in the area of inflammation by intrapulpal pressure increase, pH change, release of prostaglandins and other inflammatory mediators as well as metabolic by-products. This process is enhanced by the release of neuropeptides from nerve fibers, and thus otherwise tolerable sensations are perceived as painful.

However, it is quite possible that dentin pain results from a **direct stimulation of free nerve endings**. Recently published electron microscopic studies have demonstrated non-myelinated nerve fibers adjacent to odontoblastic processes precisely at the enamel-dentin junction.

For an understanding of the association of dental pulp pain, it is necessary to categorize according to stimulus-dependent and spontaneous pain symptoms. Spontaneous or persistent pain is indicative of advanced inflammation in the endodontium, while a reversible pulpitis can usually be successfully treated. Clinical measures targeted toward maintaining pulpal vitality are only prudent and reasonable if the pain is stimulus dependent and if the pain elicited by stimulus is of short duration.

Dentin Pain

Theories continue to be debated:

- Most well known is the *hydrodynamic theory* developed by Brännström (lower right) involving fluid movement within the dentinal tubuli.
- On the other hand, R.M. Frank and coworkers favor a *direct nerve stimulation* at the enamel-dentin junction (lower left). After special fixation with liquid nitrogen, it was possible to demonstrate non-myelinated nerve fibers in contact with odontoblastic processes at the enamel-dentin junction.

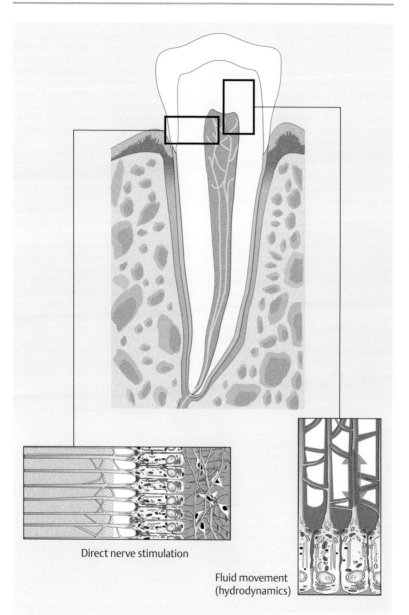

Direct nerve stimulation

Fluid movement
(hydrodynamics)

Identification of the involved tooth will demand careful evaluation of the patient's **dental history** and **clinical data collection**. The patient must be asked several important questions: When and under what conditions did the pain first occur? How long did the pain last? What triggered the pain, or did it occur spontaneously? Which tooth is involved?

It is frequently the case, however, that the patient cannot precisely identify the painful tooth. Usually the patient can only tell which side of the mouth is painful, often without cognizance of whether the pain is emanating from the maxilla or mandible.

In addition to **extraoral and intraoral clinical examinations**, sensitivity testing and percussion testing are important for identifying the involved tooth. **Sensitivity testing** can be performed electrically or thermally (see p. 34). Nevertheless, even these tests can be plagued by false-positive results, leading to identification of an incorrect tooth. A **false-positive reaction** can occur due to stimulation of periodontal ligament nerve receptors, or stimulation of the adjacent tooth if metal restorations in both teeth are in contact, as well as by improper responses on the part of the patient, who is usually already apprehensive. **False-negative results** often occur when attempting to test crowned teeth, or if the tooth surface is wet during the electrical test, or deciduous teeth or teeth whose root formation is not yet complete, and finally also in teeth that have undergone acute trauma.

Reading individual pain threshold levels on the numerical scale of an electrical sensitivity test is without diagnostic significance. However, at very high values, an additional thermal test is indicated. This should be performed using dry ice. Possible sources of error should be lower with this test in comparison to the electric sensitivity test. A heat test using warmed gutta percha is not routinely recommended, because it can lead even in a healthy tooth to irreversible pulpal damage. For a more precise localization of the involved tooth, a warmed gutta percha point may be helpful, because teeth with pulpitis react more quickly to heat.

An additional method for identification of the involved tooth involves isolation of each tooth in a quadrant using the rubber dam during the sensitivity testing. In most cases, a short waiting period must be observed from tooth-to-tooth when using the cold test.

The **percussion test** can provide supportive data concerning the periapical involvement of the involved tooth, thus improving identification. A tooth responds positively to the percussion test not only in cases of apical periodontitis but also following periodontal trauma, periodontal abscess, infraction, or tooth fracture. If numerous maxillary teeth respond positively to the percussion test, this may be a symptom of maxillary sinusitis.

Percussion and sensitivity tests should not be performed only on an individual tooth, but also on adjacent teeth, to provide comparative data.

If it proves impossible to identify the involved tooth using the test methods described above, use of **diagnostic local anesthesia** may provide a mechanism for identification. In order to differentiate between maxillary or mandibular pain, nerve block anesthesia can be employed. In order to differentiate between individual adjacent teeth, intraligamental anesthesia can be helpful. This procedure usually only reduces the sensitivity, but usually makes it possible to better target the source of the pain.

Unlocalizable pulpitic pain presents the dentist with the most difficult diagnostic demands. If the radiograph does not provide sufficient evidence, it may be necessary to simply "wait and see" until the patient's symptoms can be identified as concentrated to a single tooth.

Case Presentation

A Despite root canal treatment of the first molar, with four root canals, the severe pain experienced by the patient before treatment did not subside.

B Despite retreatment and placement of a Ledermix dressing, the pain persisted.

C The pain did not subside even after placing a Calxyl dressing.

D Only after performing root canal treatment on the *second* molar did the pain subside.

E/F After the Calxyl treatment, the root canals could be filled, and remained symptom-free.

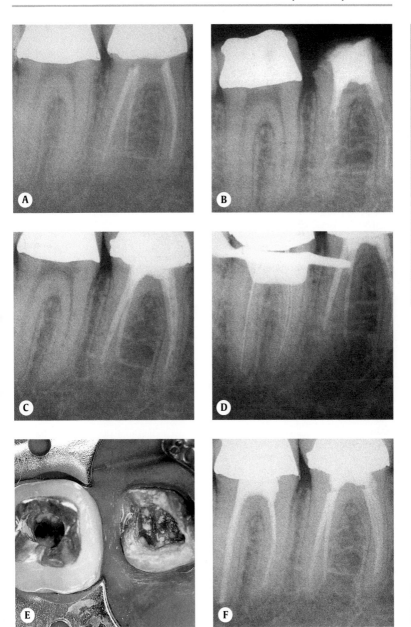

Overlooked primary root canals or apical ramifications are usually the cause of endodontic failure.

About 40% of mandibular incisors exhibit two root canals, but only in 1% does one observe two separate apical foramina. During endodontic retreatment, orthoradial and excentric radiograph projections must be made in order to depict the anatomic variations.

Approximately 84% of maxillary first premolars and ca. 58% of second premolars exhibit an additional root canal. In addition, 8% of first premolars have three or more primary ramifications.

During embryologic development, the mesiobuccal and the mesiopalatal root canals of the maxillary first molars share a common primary root canal. During tooth development, invagination and the deposition of hard tissue occur, so that the palatal segment in the mesiobuccal root becomes smaller and may even be partially or completely obliterated.

The most probable cause for endodontic failure in maxillary molars is insufficient instrumentation with untreated canals and foramina.

Mandibular premolars exhibit the most complicated root canal system. Approximately 31% of first premolars and 11% of second premolars exhibit two ramifications, and 3% have even a third **primary** canal.

The root canals must be probed using fine, prebent files (size 10). The file is inserted along the outer wall of the already localized canal until resistance or a diversion is encountered. Using slight rotatory movements, the final extent of the canal is completely traversed.

Secondary and tertiary ramifications are branches of the primary root canal, lateral or accessory canals that open into the periodontal ligament space. More than 20% of all anterior teeth and 50% of posterior teeth exhibit numerous ramifications. These branches are virtually impossible to instrument mechanically, but copious rinsing with sodium hypochlorite solution is effective for cleaning. During retreatment, these ramifications are usually closed with paste or dentin chips, so the complete removal of tissue is not possible.

The opening into the pulp chamber must provide uninhibited access and vision into the pulp chamber. A rubber dam should always be placed before opening the pulp chamber. All carious dentin must be excavated and overlying tooth hard structure removed appropriately. The size and depth of the pulp chamber should be measured with the help of radiographs. The removal of cervical ledges is of particular importance for the identification of additional canals. This also simplifies access to dilacerated canals. If the additional canals are not localized and identified, postoperative pain, swelling or even fistula formation may occur.

Case Presentation

A Missed canal: The maxillary second premolar following trepanation and debridement and filling of the root canal exhibits a **second** root canal that was not initially observed. Following the initial endodontic treatment, the patient complained of spontaneously occurring severe pain, but the dentist did not elect to retreat the case.

B The diagnostic radiograph reveals a periapical radiolucency despite an apparently successful root canal filling; the filling, however, did not extend to the apex because of the severe dilaceration of the canal.

C The second root canal was instrumented completely to the apical constriction, and the original filling of the first canal was left in place because it appeared radiographically to be well adapted.

D Three months after placement of a Calxyl temporary dressing, the second canal was thoroughly rinsed and the canal was filled with gutta percha. Initial regeneration of the periapical radiolucency is visible.

E Two months later, the tooth was prosthetically restored following placement of two screw-type posts in the root canal.

F One year after retreatment, the periapical radiolucency has completely disappeared, and the tooth was treated with a full crown.

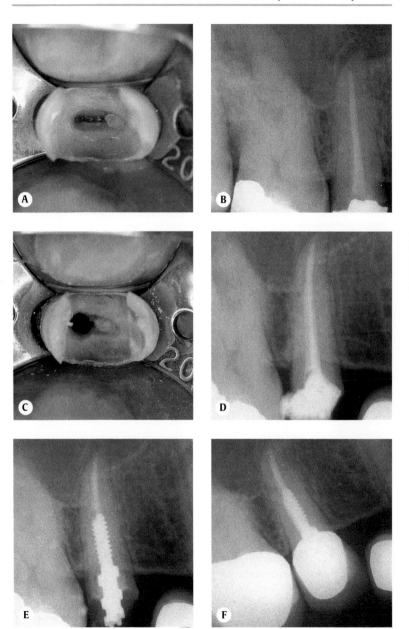

Crown infractions are actually quite common, and appear as lines within the enamel; but they usually do not extend beyond this. Infractions are usually only the result of tooth trauma, but may also be combined with other injuries such as tooth luxation.

Usually, pure crown infractions require **no treatment**. However, because of the frequent occurrence of attendant injury to the tooth-supporting apparatus, **sensitivity tests** should be performed to ascertain the possibility of pulpal injury.

Infractions in posterior teeth are incomplete fractures that occur in both restored and sound teeth. They normally course **vertically**, and a horizontal infraction is less common. Vertical infractions course through the posterior tooth crown in the mesiodistal direction, and may involve one or both proximal surfaces.

Crown infractions occur most frequently in mandibular first molars and maxillary premolars.

Etiologic factors include all situations that reduce the stability of the tooth, e.g., parafunctions, masticatory trauma, expansive caries, parapulpal pin retention, and poorly configured cavity preparations.

The **clinical symptoms** depend upon the depth of the infraction. With superficial infractions, pain is relatively seldom. In many patients, pain is experienced during mastication, especially when pressure on the tooth is released. Deep infractions that extend even to the pulp chamber exhibit symptoms of an acute, irreversible pulpitis. Crown infraction is not characterized by any certain clinical symptom, but rather by a myriad of vague discomforts.

The affected region is first carefully inspected with magnification loupes, cold light, as well as the electric caries meter. In questionable cases, the occlusal region is stained using methylene blue. These techniques, however, do not permit a precise determination of the extent, depth, and course of the infraction. After ruling out other etiologies, the patient should be asked to quickly tap the teeth together repeatedly. Pain that occurs following release of occlusal biting force indicates an incomplete vertical fracture.

Following dental trauma without any loss of tooth hard structure, changes in color, tooth mobility and luxation should be observed, and both thermal and electric sensitivity tests should be performed. Shortly following trauma, tooth color can change and the sensitivity test may be negative. Gradually, the tooth color and sensitivity often return to that of a normal tooth. In such cases, no clinical treatment is indicated. The patient should be examined every six months, because of the possibility of calcification within the root canal.

If pain occurs following infraction, it must be assumed that the infraction is deep, that it has penetrated into dentin and has reached the pulpal tissues. The first therapeutic measure is **stabilization of the crown**, which can be accomplished in the posterior segments by steel or copper bands, and in the anterior teeth by means of adhesive restorations or a temporary crown.

If pulpitis is diagnosed, the tooth must be opened and endodontic treatment performed. The root canals should not be excessively widened. If the tooth remains symptom-free following placement of temporary dressings, the root canals are filled with thermoplastic gutta percha. Complications following endodontic treatment may occur independent of the technique employed.

Adhesive cements and composite materials are then used to close the coronal opening in the tooth. The definitive restoration should be an onlay or a crown.

Case Presentation

A In the radiograph, the painful, crowned mandibular second molar exhibits a periapical radiolucency.

B Following removal of the crown and the caries, a fracture is visible at the floor of the cavity.

C This is a line of infraction.

D The distal perforation was closed, the root canals were instrumented and rinsed. The fracture line is clearly visible in the surgical microscope.

E The root canals were carefully filled using thermoplastic gutta percha.

F Radiograph following definitive endodontic therapy.

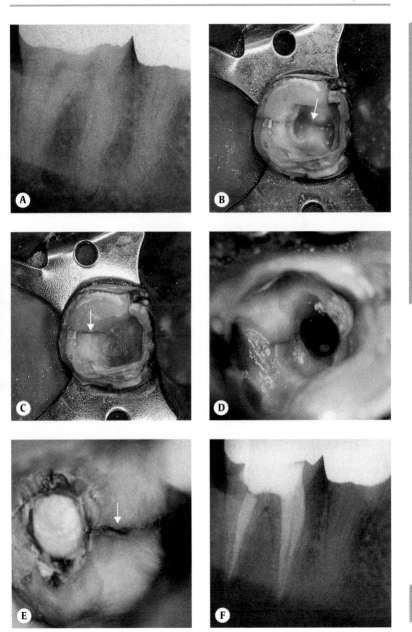

Injuries to teeth should always be considered as **emergencies**. After the following types of dental injury, pulpal necrosis occurs in the percentages listed:

- enamel fracture · · · · · · · · · · · · · · · 1%
- enamel-dentin fracture · · · · · · · · · 3%
- complicated crown fracture with pulp exposure · · · · · · · · · · · · 4%
- root fracture · · · · · · · · · · · · · · · · · · 20%
- lateral luxation · · · · · · · · · · · · · · · 58%
- intrusion · 85%.

Extra-alveolar crown fractures can be classified as **uncomplicated and without pulp exposure** and **complicated fracture with pulp exposure**. Treatment will be determined by the stage of the tooth root development and the expected pulpal reaction. Depending upon the expanse of the fracture site, it can be closed and built-up using composite resin (total bonding). Radiographs taken six months afterwards and later at annual intervals will reveal any pathologic mineralization or periapical lesions that might require endodontic treatment.

In the case of complicated crown fracture, the pulpal tissues are exposed after dentin destruction. Depending upon the extent of destruction, emergency treatment may involve direct pulp capping or vital amputation. A subsequent complete endodontic treatment is recommended. A success rate of 90% can be expected following direct pulp capping, with formation of a hard tissue bridge of secondary dentin; the results are better with incomplete root formation (94%) compared with completely formed roots (88%).

Pulp amputation 2 mm subjacent to the exposure was successful in 90% of young patients, independent of the localization and size of the pulp exposure as well as the time of treatment.

With complete crown fracture, failure to treat the exposed pulp will lead to necrosis over the long term. The **stage of development** is of critical significance for the choice of therapy. In young teeth with incomplete root growth, an exposed pulp should be maintained, while in teeth with complete root formation the pulp should be removed.

In the absence of clinical symptoms or radiographic periapical reactions on teeth with advanced root formation, treatment success

can be expected. However, fully one-quarter of traumatically damaged teeth may develop obliteration of the root canal within four years, providing an indication for timely endodontic therapy even in the absence of clinical symptoms.

Failure to treat initial pulp exposure for more than one month after trauma led to a 100% incidence of necrosis of the pulpal tissue. In addition, apical periodontitis also developed. Even in cases of enamel-dentin fractures without pulp exposure, over 50% of patients exhibited tissue necrosis and in about 7% extreme root resorption.

If pain persists after treatment of the crown fracture by means of composite resin build-up, the pulp must be extirpated, and the definitive restoration can be placed at the same appointment. If over time necrosis and apical periodontitis occur, the root canal must be instrumented and a temporary calcium hydroxide dressing placed.

Case Presentation

A Maxillary central incisor fracture in a 13-year-old patient without pulp exposure. No treatment for this tooth was performed for seven days. An acute, irreversible pulpitis ensued.

B The radiograph depicted no periapical lesion, the apical foramen was still wide open, and the tooth did not respond to a sensitivity test.

C Using infiltration anesthesia, the pulp was extirpated and the root canal was carefully and copiously rinsed with 5% sodium hypochlorite.

D Using the radiograph, the working length was established such that the root canal was instrumented up to ca. 1 mm short of the apical foramen.

E Two weeks later, the loose Calxyl dressing was removed with a K file and calcium hydroxide was inserted.

F One year later, additional root development was observed; the gutta percha main point was carefully measured.

G/H Filling of the root canal and follow-up radiograph.

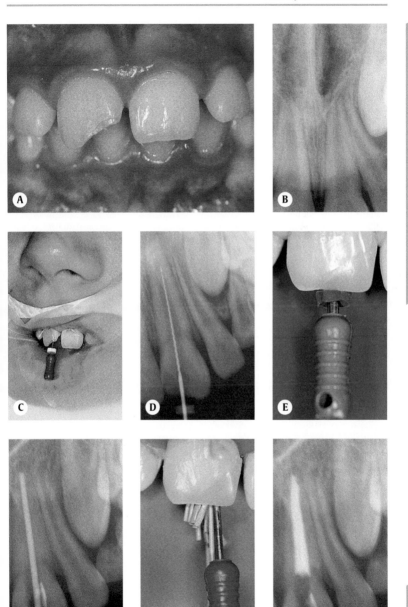

Root fractures represent combined injury to dentin, cementum, pulp, and periodontal tissue. Fractures in the apical and middle third are usually oblique. A frontal impact dislodges the coronal fragment palatally and slightly out of the alveolus.

Root fractures are usually associated with other dental injuries: Fracture of the alveolar process is also frequently observed. Clinical examination usually reveals **extrusion** of the tooth, frequently with lingual (palatal) displacement.

It is usually no problem to detect the obliquely coursing fracture in the **radiograph**. Nevertheless, it is prudent to take two additional films with a deviation of at least 15° from the plane of the fracture. The root fracture can occur in the middle or apical third of the root. In most cases, a single, obliquely coursing line indicating the fracture is visible on the radiograph. However, there may also be multiple fractures or the fracture line may be ellipsoid and give a false impression of multiple fractures.

Four **healing processes** may occur following root fracture:

- healing via calcified tissue: a callus of hard tissue unites the fracture
- interposition of connective tissue between the root fragments, often partially or completely obliterating the root canal
- interposition of bone and connective tissue with normal periodontal ligament around the fragments
- the appearance of inflammatory granulation tissue.

Stable fixation is the basis for treatment success. Fractures in the middle third of the root without dislocation of the crown should be splinted for six to eight weeks. In young patients, it is possible to maintain pulpal vitality. With sufficiently stable fixation of the tooth, there will be connective tissue repair or even mineralized bridging of the fracture line. The tooth must be evaluated radiographically and via sensitivity tests in order to provide early diagnosis of pulpal necrosis.

In cases of dislocation, the root fragment bearing the crown must be repositioned and splinted. If the radiograph provides evidence of radiolucency or resorption, indicating pulp

necrosis, the root canal must be debrided, instrumented, and temporarily filled with calcium hydroxide. Because the apical root fragment is usually vital, root canal treatment is necessary only in the coronal fragment. Alternatively, it may be possible to connect the two fragments via a post construction. In some patients, the apical root fragment must be removed.

A vertical, perpendicularly oriented root fracture involves the crown and root, and usually affects also the root canal. Enhancing factors include weakening of the root structure due to expansive canal instrumentation, as well as mechanically unfavorable placement of screws and post build-ups.

The clinical diagnosis is difficult because there are no clear clinical symptoms of root fracture. In 95% of patients, periodontal pockets may occur, dull pain sensation occurs in 66%, periodontal abscess in 28% and fistula in 13%. Additional **clinical signs** are osseous defects, pus release, swelling and tooth mobility.

The goal of **therapy** is elimination of the fracture gap, through which a communication with the oral cavity is created. Single-rooted teeth are usually extracted; with multirooted teeth, the affected root may be hemisected.

Case Presentation

A Vertical root fracture of the mesial root one week after root canal instrumentation.

B Clinically, the crown is obviously fractured and the mesial segment is mobile.

C The distal root canal is instrumented and filled, following placement of an interim dressing.

D The crown is sectioned buccolingually, leaving more tooth structure on the distal segment.

E Following hemisection, the mesial half of the tooth is carefully extracted.

F The screw is seated without tension.

G The missing half of the molar is replaced with a bridge pontic.

H Radiograph immediately after seating the bridge.

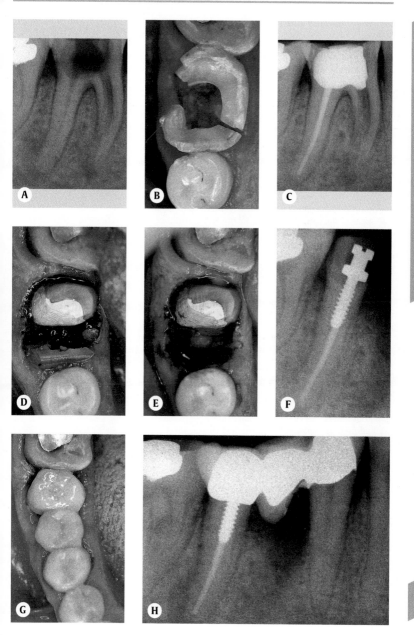

The concept of direct pulp capping involves covering an exposed pulp with a wound dressing that protects the pulpal tissue from additional injury. An inflammation-free pulp that is inadvertently exposed during tooth preparation will exhibit a high degree of regenerative potential. Any hemorrhage must be staunched using a sterile cotton pellet because a blood coagulum between the pulp and the capping material can reduce the rate of healing by about 50%.

The condition of the pulp at the very time of exposure is critical for success. An **inflammation-free pulp** possesses a high **regeneration potential**, which decreases with increasing severity of inflammation. If the exposed pulp tissue is contaminated by bacteria before placement of the capping material, failure is the rule. On the other hand, it is questionable whether clinical examination can always lead to a correct diagnosis of the severity of inflammation within the pulp. The absolute prerequisite for success of direct pulp capping is an inflammation-free pulp.

The expanse of the exposure appears to be of less significance than the location of the exposure.

Clinical studies have reported extremely variable **success rates after direct pulp capping**, ranging from 97.8% after 1.5 years, and dropping to 61.4% after five years. As reported in a recently published study, the clinical-radiographic success fell from 37% at five years to only 13% after 10 years. Comparable clinical studies of immediate vital extirpation of the exposed pulp demonstrated a clearly higher rate of success: For example, the success rate of all endodontically treated teeth in the private practice of Rocke revealed 93% success after five years and 81% after 10 years. Such results present a clear indication for immediate endodontic therapy with extirpation of pulpal tissues and canal instrumentation, even if only a tiny pulp exposure occurs.

An **exception** to this general rule is pulp exposure in a tooth whose **root formation is yet incomplete**. Direct pulp capping in a permanent tooth with incomplete root development consists of covering the exposed pulp with a wound dressing that induces the formation of new hard tissue. If the exposure is contaminated by bacteria from dental caries or through contact with saliva over 24 hours, successful treatment cannot be expected.

The most intense Ca^{2+}-release and therefore the greatest inductive stimulation for hard tissue formation is elicited by aqueous calcium hydroxide preparations; however, the calcium necessary for formation of the hard tissue bridge does not derive from $Ca(OH)_2$, but rather from the body's own tissue.

Beneath the $Ca(OH)_2$-induced three-layered tissue necrosis, one observes differentiation of secondary odontoblasts, and in the most favorable case, an irregular osteoid-like secondary dentin is formed.

Recent studies report good results after use of mineral trioxide (MTA), as well as the use of calcitonin, collagen, zinc oxide-eugenol (ZnOE), or dentin bonding and composite resin.

Case Presentation

A Immediately after pulp exposure, hemorrhage must be staunched.

B The carious process has not yet reached the pulp.

C Aqueous $Ca(OH)_2$ (e.g., Calxyl red) is painted thinly and carefully onto the exposure using a sterile cotton pellet. Care should be taken to avoid any possible subsequent hemorrhagic leaking. If this becomes visible, the capping material must be rinsed away and placed again after hemorrhage is completely stopped. Excessive capping material is removed carefully with an excavator, leaving only the perforation site covered.

D The pulp capping material must be placed only onto caries-free dentin.

E The calcium hydroxide is covered with zinc oxide-eugenol, and subsequently with phosphate or glass ionomer cement, and a definitive restoration using composite resin.

F Immediately adjacent to the regeneratively inflamed pulp (5) with temporarily limited injury, one observes reparative dentin (2), a diffuse mineralization (3), osteoid dentin (4) and the zone of necrosis (5). The calcium hydroxide (1) is covered with ZnOE, and this is then covered by glass ionomer cement and a composite resin restoration (total bonding).

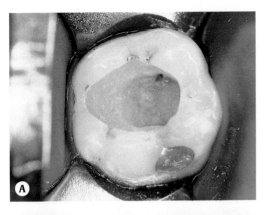

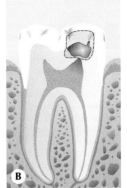

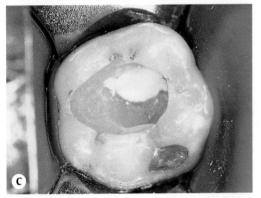

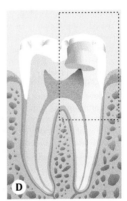

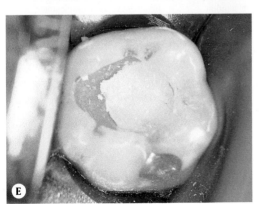

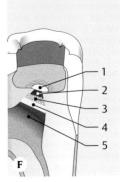

1
2
3
4
5

53

The indication for pulpotomy on a symptom-free permanent tooth exhibiting incomplete root development is a broad pulp exposure with or without inflammation limited to the coronal pulp.

The time between pulp exposure (e.g., trauma) to treatment should not exceed 48 hours.

A differentiation is made between a **partial pulpotomy** with removal of only some of the coronal pulp and leaving behind segments of the coronal pulp with healing potential, and a **complete pulpotomy** with removal of the entire coronal pulp. The prerequisite for partial pulpotomy is that hemorrhage can be completely stopped within five minutes after removal of pulpal tissue. If hemorrhage persists beyond this time, complete pulpal amputation should be performed.

Pulpal amputation is an **interim procedure**. In addition to the formation of a hard tissue bridge, even after only four months one may observe island-like deposition of secondary dentin, which can lead to almost complete obliteration of the root canal. Following completion of root development, root canal therapy including extirpation of the remaining pulp should be performed even if the patient is symptom-free.

The goal of pulpotomy is therefore a time-limited **vital maintenance** of the root canal pulp. This should guarantee completion of root development and the formation of an apical constriction.

Under local anesthesia, the coronal pulp is removed using a high-speed diamond bur, the pulp chamber is rinsed with saline solution, and a sterile cotton pellet is used to staunch any hemorrhage by applying pressure onto the root canal orifices. A blood coagulum between the pulp capping material and the residual root canal pulp will delay or inhibit the formation of a hard tissue bridge.

A thin layer of calcium hydroxide is applied, and then checked for any hemorrhagic oozing; then additional calcium hydroxide to a thickness of 2 mm is applied, and covered by IRM and also a layer of glass ionomer cement.

For **pulp capping** in young permanent teeth, calcium hydroxide is the material of choice. A mixture of tricalcium phosphate (TCP) induces hard tissue formation without causing tissue destruction in adjacent pulp

tissue that is typical for pure calcium hydroxide. A tight coronal closure appears to be equally important for clinical success.

At regular three to six month follow-up appointments, the success of therapy is appraised clinically and root development is checked radiographically. Sensitivity tests on pulp-amputated teeth are of little significance.

In a clinical study of 37 permanent teeth, treatment success was achieved in 93.5% of patients without clinical or radiographic symptoms; however, for symptomatic teeth with periapical lesions, pulpotomy can also be completely successful.

In the deciduous dentition, pulpal amputation is preferable to pulp capping for exposed vital tissue. After removal of the coronal pulp, hemorrhage can be stopped using a sterile cotton pellet saturated with ferrous sulfate. If bleeding stops following removal of the pellet, the amputation site is covered with zinc oxide-eugenol cement. Additional treatment includes coverage with a glass ionomer cement and a composite resin restoration.

Case Presentation

A The bitewing radiograph of the left posterior segment in a 13-year-old female reveals deep caries on the mesial of tooth 36.

B During caries excavation, an expansive exposure of the pulp occurred. As a temporary measure, the coronal pulp was extirpated.

C Using the radiograph, the root development was determined at the initiation of endodontic treatment. If root development is well progressed, the pulpotomy can be viewed as a short-term solution lasting until completion of root formation.

D Using a high-speed diamond bur, the coronal pulp tissue is removed to the level of the root canal orifices.

E Application of a sterile cotton pellet to staunch any hemorrhage.

F Calcium hydroxide in an aqueous suspension is painted in a thin layer over the pulp stumps, and checked carefully for hemorrhagic oozing. Subsequently the calcium hydroxide layer is increased to a thickness of 1–2 mm and the cavity is tightly closed with an appropriate restorative material.

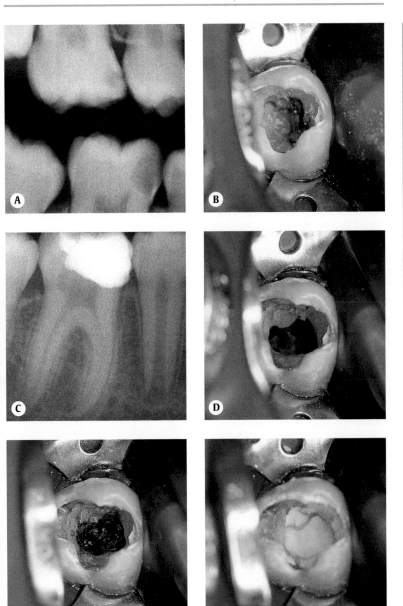

The diagnosis and treatment of painful diseases of the pulp present the general dental practitioner with problems, because these patients will be significantly influenced and confused by their pain. In addition, the dentist is also often confronted with a dental history and clinical findings that do not permit precise classification of the inflammatory condition. If the patient is able to precisely identify the painful tooth, and if the radiograph clearly depicts a pathologic condition, or if clinical symptoms such as percussion sensitivity or a fistula point to the involved tooth as well as to the general pathophysiological situation, a rapid decision concerning treatment can be made. On the other hand, if the patient experiences radiating, diffuse pain without any clear identification of a particular tooth, treatment must begin only symptomatically.

An **irreversible pulpitis** may be characterized by a wide variety of clinical symptoms:

- pain that persists beyond the stimulation
- pain elicited more by heat than by cold
- radiating pain, including spontaneously occurring pain with pulse synchrony.

For emergency treatment of irreversible pulpitis, **a careful endodontic treatment with extirpation and temporary restoration** has the highest success rate, with 99% freedom from pain. Especially with molar teeth, however, this procedure is usually not performable as an unplanned therapy. Nevertheless, the goal must be immediate relief of the patient's pain, and this can be quickly accomplished even with multirooted teeth without the use of toxic medicaments and with the option of performing a well-planned comprehensive root canal treatment later.

To relieve pain, the method of choice is **amputation of the coronal pulp** to the level of the root canal orifices. With a success rate of 96%, this technique is equivalent to the more time-consuming vital extirpation with complete instrumentation of the root canal.

With the rubber dam in place and with local anesthesia, a high-speed bur is used to completely remove caries, and subsequently, after changing the bur, high speed is also used to remove the coronal pulp. Using a moist, sterile cotton pellet, any hemorrhage is staunched, a eugenol-soaked cotton pellet is applied, and the tooth is closed using Cavit.

The use of chlorophenol camphor, Cresatin, zinc oxide-eugenol (ZnOE), and saline solution can also be employed, as well as the application of a dry cotton pellet. In one clinical study, 78% of patients so treated were completely free of pain after the anesthesia wore off. Topical application of corticosteroids will also lead to freedom from symptoms, but simultaneously the regenerative capabilities of the pulp are reduced. Histologically, the picture is usually one of chronic forms of inflammation. Eugenol's first effect is one of anesthesia, and secondly a reduction of prostaglandin synthesis, which reduces inflammation but can also be neurotoxic.

Case Presentation

A Mandibular first premolar exhibited persistent pain to heat and after eating; note the advanced distal proximal carious lesion.

B Under local anesthesia the coronal pulp was excavated, and a sterile cotton pellet was used to stop hemorrhage.

C The crown preparation was performed using a high-speed diamond, and the pulp was removed up to the level of the entrances to the root canals.

D Following hemostasis, either a dry or a eugenol-saturated cotton pellet was pressed onto the canal orifices, and the cavity was subsequently sealed with a temporary restoration.

E/F One week following emergency treatment, the root canals were instrumented.

G A calcium hydroxide interim dressing was left in place for three weeks, and then the canals were definitively filled.

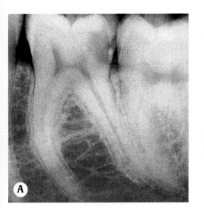

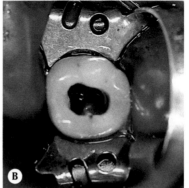

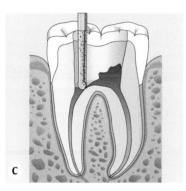

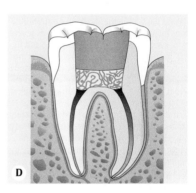

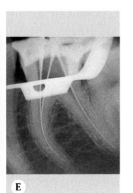

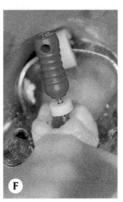

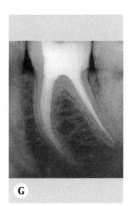

57

Emergency treatment in the deciduous dentition, including treatment for pulp exposure, is different from treatment for permanent teeth because **direct pulp capping** has a less favorable prognosis, and therefore pulpal amputation is the treatment of choice. However, if the pulp exposure is very small and there is no indication of pulpitic changes, an attempt at direct pulp capping may be justified. Nevertheless, if the pulp exposure occurs in carious dentin or if pulpal damage has already occurred, **pulpotomy** or **vital amputation** is always is the treatment of choice. Pulpotomy includes the total amputation of the coronal pulp up to the root canal orifices.

Amputation is **indicated** following simple or multiple exposures of the vital deciduous tooth pulp. In cases of traumatic pulp exposure, the amputation can still be performed several days after the incident. **Contraindications** include clinical symptoms such as severe pain, swelling, percussion sensitivity, and fistula formation, as well as elevated tooth mobility. Radiographic contraindications include changes such as internal and/or advanced external root resorption, as well as periapical and intraradicular lesions.

Today, the pulpotomy procedure is mainly limited to vital deciduous teeth. The primary goal is relief of pain and the limited maintenance of the tooth if no disadvantageous reactions are expected in the adjacent teeth, permanent teeth or the general health of the patient. These goals will be achieved following complete removal of the inflamed tissues as well as the application of an impermeable cavity closure.

Local anesthesia must be administered before **amputation** in cases of vital pulp exposure. The coronal pulp is removed using a high-speed diamond bur under constant saline irrigation; this will provide the best possible control of hemorrhage. After complete removal of all soft tissues, and thorough rinsing of the area, a sterile cotton pellet is pressed into the cavity to stop bleeding. Subsequently the pulp-capping material is applied and the tooth is securely closed coronally.

If **hemostasis** is inadequate, a blood coagulum forms, which can lead to chronic inflammation and subsequent internal root resorption. Hemostasis can be enhanced or supported by the application of a cotton pellet saturated with **ferrous sulfate solution**, aluminum chloride, or vasoconstrictors such as adrenalin. Ferrous sulfate solution (15.5%) combined with a zinc oxide-eugenol filling led to an almost 100% success rate after two years. Electrosurgery and lasers may also be used for hemostasis.

Following the application of calcium hydroxide in the vital procedure in deciduous teeth, the formation of a hard tissue bridge may occur. Clinical studies indicate a success rate of 31–100% of treated teeth, histologically, however, only 50% exhibit a dentin bridge and healing, the remainder show inflammation and resorption.

Still today, **formocresol**, a combination of 19% formaldehyde and 35% cresol, is used in the deciduous dentition. Application for five minutes leads to superficial fixation, and in adjacent areas one observes vital but chronically inflamed pulpal tissue. In such cases, pure zinc oxide-eugenol is applied to the amputated tissue and the tooth is securely closed. The systemic distribution of formocresol within the organism represents a negative concern, despite the clinical success rate of 94–98% in the deciduous dentition.

Case Presentation

A A high-speed bur is used to remove the coronal pulp tissue and to completely clean the entire cavity.

B Vital pulp tissue is removed to the level of the root canal orifices.

C Hemorrhage control is enhanced by a ferrous sulfate-saturated cotton pellet.

D The cotton pellet is pressed into the cavity for five minutes and then removed.

E Following hemorrhage control, the amputation site is covered with zinc oxide-eugenol cement without additional ingredients. This layer is then covered with glass ionomer cement.

F The coronal aspect of the cavity is finally filled using composite resin.

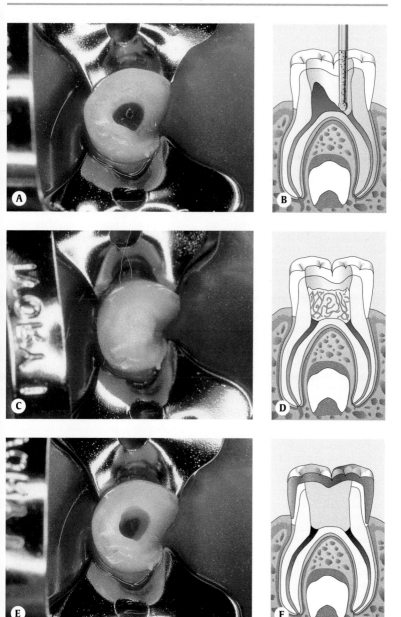

Endodontic therapy is indicated in deciduous teeth with irreversible pulpitis or necrosis. **Contraindications** include a nonrestorable tooth, radiographically visible internal resorption, teeth exhibiting mechanical or carious perforation of the pulp chamber floor, expansive pathologic resorption of more than one-third of the root, bone resorption with furcation involvement, as well as sharply demarcated periapical lesions. Aside from these situations, pulpectomy can be clinically successful in 96% of cases.

In the anterior segment, the trepanation opening is on the lingual aspect; in the posterior segments, the thin dentin canal floor must be carefully approached. The prebent hand instruments widen the canal 2–3 mm shorter than the radiographic length, and must not perforate the thin walls. Because the apical ramifications cannot be approached mechanically, copious rinsing with sodium hypochlorite solution must be performed. The root canals are instrumented to ca. size 35, and then a temporary $Ca(OH)_2$ dressing is placed for 10 days.

Only when the patient is completely free of pain can the root canals be definitively filled. The canals are filled using **resorbable zinc oxide-eugenol** without additives, in the nonanesthetized tooth. Nonresorbable materials such as gutta percha point are contraindicated. An exception to this general rule is deciduous teeth where no succedaneous tooth exists.

Following the endodontic therapy, the tooth crown is restored. Secure closure of the cavity must be given high priority because tight closure will prohibit bacterial recontamination and subsequent failure.

The pulpectomy procedure is very time-consuming, and therefore requires a very cooperative patient as well as understanding parents. Patient and parents must be made aware of the **risks** of endodontic therapy, including possible injury of the permanent tooth or tooth bud. Preparation of a measurement radiograph is absolutely necessary. Electronic measurement of the root canal length is not sufficiently precise in the deciduous dentition. Endodontic therapy for deciduous teeth must generally be very critically evaluated. The "cost-to-benefit ratio" must be carefully evaluated with consideration for the patient's own receptivity and also the high level of operator commitment in terms of time and effort. If the child patient is insufficiently cooperative, it may be necessary to compromise treatment procedures to eliminate pain.

Even today, the most often employed technique is to simply leave the tooth open following expansive trepanation. One can differentiate between leaving the cavity only partially open (drainage) or leaving the deciduous tooth cavity completely open. If the deciduous tooth is to be left partially open, following trepanation the cavity is partially closed so that only a canal-like access remains. If the tooth is left completely open, after trepanation the tooth is shortened to the height of the gingiva and the infected pulpal tissue is removed as far as possible. Leaving the cavity open in this way does not provide a long-term satisfactory solution, particularly with regard to motivation toward adequate oral hygiene. This is a **compromise treatment** that serves only to save some time before definitive treatment if this cannot be performed during the same appointment.

Case Presentation

A Under the rubber dam, the deciduous tooth is trephined and the coronal pulp is removed. Because the cavity floor is thinner than in a permanent tooth, the danger of perforation is high.

B Based on the diagnostic radiograph, the anticipated length is determined, and following careful instrumentation with a Hedström file the working length is determined, which is 2–3 mm short of the apex.

C Zinc oxide-eugenol without additives in a thick consistency is applied to the floor of the cavity and pressed into the root canals using a sterile cotton pellet.

D Using a graduated plugger, the root canal filling material is slowly placed into the canal, without overfilling the canal.

E Completed endodontic treatment with definitive closure of the coronal cavity.

F One and two years later, radiographs are taken to determine the success of the treatment as well as normal deciduous root resorption.

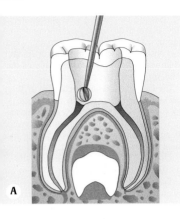

A

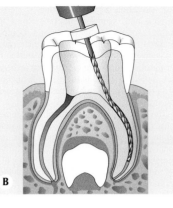

B

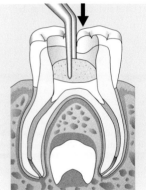

C

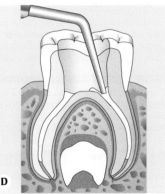

D

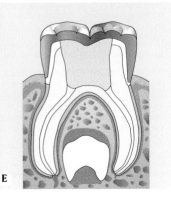

E

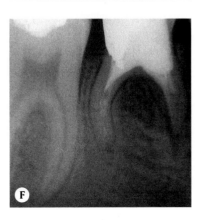

F

Emergency Treatment

The indication for **apexification** is pulpal necrosis and incomplete root development. Further root development in the face of pulpal necrosis is highly unlikely; the root canal walls diverge apically making preparation of an apical stop impossible. Treatment is therefore targeted toward inducing the formation of an apical buttress of hard tissue, and avoiding any overfilling of the canal.

The working length is established somewhat shorter in order to avoid overinstrumentation. Because of the thin dentin walls, the canal must not be excessively widened, rather copious rinsing with sodium hypochlorite in a 5% concentration is performed. This provides additional chemical tissue dissolution. If apically open root canals are treated with calcium hydroxide for three to six months with a dressing change every four weeks, the result is resolution of the periapical inflammation and the **formation of cementoid hard substance**. If the root canals are not filled with calcium hydroxide, the inflammation persists and no apical closure occurs.

For **apical closure**, collagen preparations, calcium phosphate as well as more recently mineral trioxide (MTA, "ProRoot") is recommended. According to experimental studies and early clinical results, MTA appears to be equal to a calcium hydroxide closure, and a long-term dressing is not necessary.

One of the most important factors for success in addition to complete debridement and removal of all necrotic tissue remnants is an impermeable closure of the coronal cavity to prevent new immigration of microorganisms.

If the root canal is to be treated with calcium hydroxide dressings, it must be first thoroughly cleansed. The working length is determined using the radiograph and is established 1–2 mm shorter. Electronic length determination is unreliable in teeth with incomplete root development. Traumatization of the apical tissues must be avoided during canal instrumentation, because it is from the cells in the periapical region that hard tissue formation will derive.

After final rinsing and drying of the canal, calcium hydroxide powder is mixed with physiologic saline and placed into the root canals using paper points of appropriate length. Because the diameter of the canals is large,

one can use the paper points upside down. The calcium hydroxide is carefully condensed into the canal using a dry paper point, which also absorbs any excessive fluid. Thereafter, additional calcium hydroxide is placed and condensed with a dry paper point.

The $Ca(OH)_2$ dressing is changed at three weeks and after three months, and remains in the root canal for about one year. The formation of a hard tissue bridge requires between six months and two years. Thereafter, the root canal can be definitively filled. Several gutta percha points are placed into eucalyptus oil for about four seconds in order to soften the surface. Thereafter, upon a sterile glass slab, a mixing spatula is used to shape an appropriate gutta percha point to the diameter of the canal. This shaped point is inserted into the moist canal and seated using a sealer.

Case Presentation

A Symptom-free maxillary incisor in a 14-year-old patient, exhibiting a vestibular fistula and a likely traumatic enamel defect.

B The radiograph depicts the periapical lesion and the wide-open apical foramen.

C For apexification, the entire root canal is filled with calcium hydroxide. ZnOE and a temporary restoration close the coronal cavity.

D Following calcium hydroxide treatment, a hard substance bridge has formed apically.

E If MTA is to be used to fill the canal, the canal must first be thoroughly rinsed and dried. Using a plugger, the MTA is inserted into the apical canal region in 3-mm layer thicknesses. The canal can then be immediately obturated with gutta percha.

F After three months of Calxyl, the periapical lesion is significantly reduced in size.

G One year later, the canal can be definitively filled with gutta percha.

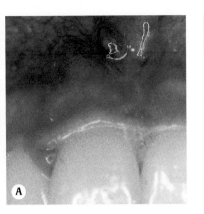

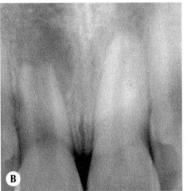

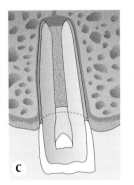

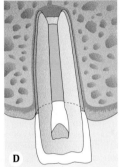

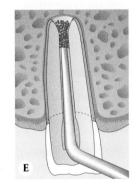

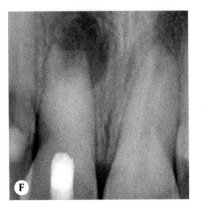

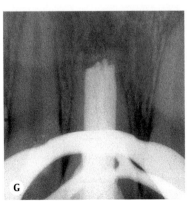

In a study of teeth with apical periodontitis, the size of the periapical lesion correlated with the expanse of bacterial invasion and the tissue destruction within the root canal pulp. Teeth exhibiting a large periapical radiolucency no longer responded to a thermal sensitivity test. With small apical radiolucencies, the teeth still responded positively. Histologically, tissue necrosis was limited to the coronal pulp. The tissue in the apical segments of the root canal was fully intact and free of any accumulation of inflammatory cells. Thus, **periapical lesions** develop long before a **total pulpitis** ensues, likely due to the penetration of endotoxins that are released from the outer membranes of gram-negative bacteria upon their death. In addition, even in severely inflamed areas of the pulp, **intact nerve fibers** can be seen in the electron microscope.

The goal of **emergency treatment** in cases of pulpal tissue necrosis is relief of pain, without completely instrumenting the root canal. In contrast to irreversible pulpitis, the diagnosis is usually simplified by the fact that the radiograph already reveals an initial periapical radiolucency.

In contrast to the treatment of irreversible pulpitis, the necrotic pulpal tissue must be removed from the root canals even if such removal is not complete, as long as it extends to the transition into the apical third of the canal. The **chances for success** are optimum if, during the initial appointment, the root canals can be completely instrumented, which is normally possible with single-rooted teeth. With multirooted posterior teeth, it is often difficult to achieve freedom from pain within 20 minutes by complete cleaning/instrumentation of all root canals, due to the root canal anatomy.

Because the greatest concentration of bacteria in the necrotically involved coronal pulp is located at or near the transition to the coronal root canal pulp, the goal of emergency therapy is to completely remove this area of inflamed tissue, therefore eliminating the source of the patient's pain. This is performed exclusively using the crown-down technique, in which the procedure is initiated coronally and proceeds apically. Best success will be achieved with excellent coronal access. Subsequently, Gates–Glidden drills, starting with sizes 4 or 5, are used to widen the canal orifices. Very important is thorough rinsing with 5% sodium hypochlorite solution and the use of a lubricant (e.g., Glyde, RC prep, Calcinase-Slide). Using a small Gates drill, progression is made deeper into the root canal. Subsequently a Nitinol instrument of conicity 6 (e.g., Flexmaster 0.06, Profile 0.06) and 21-mm length, size 25 or 30, achieves the coronal and middle thirds of the root canal, without penetrating into the apical 3–4 mm, because vital tissue remains in this region. The instrumented canals are again copiously rinsed and then closed using Cavit. In patients who cannot be comprehensively treated within three to five days, the root canals may be filled with Ledermix. Otherwise only the rinsing solution remains in the canal.

Case Presentation

A–C An **alternative emergency treatment** for multirooted teeth is the complete instrumentation of only the largest root canal (e.g., maxillary palatal canal). The other narrow and dilacerated canals are not instrumented at all despite the presence of necrotic material. For this treatment, Gates drills are used initially to remove the main mass of necrotic material coronally.

D After radiographic determination of the working length, the root canal is completely instrumented to the apex. A Lentulo spiral can be used to rotate in an interim dressing of Calxyl; then the trepanation opening is closed at its coronal aspect.

E/F Five days later, the other two canals are completely instrumented and the working lengths determined radiographically. The interim dressing is Calxyl, applied using paper points.

G Four weeks later, the dressing is removed, the canals are rinsed and dried.

H If the patient is symptom-free, definitive root canal filling can be performed.

I Radiograph of the definitive root canal filling.

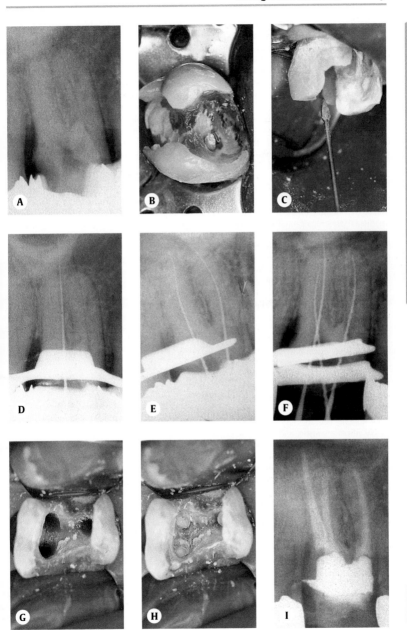

The American Association of Endodontists defines a "flare up" as an **acute exacerbation** of a periapical inflammation following initiation of or during endodontic treatment. The incidence of such postoperative pain varies according to various studies between 1.4% and 45%, and in most patients necessitates an additional appointment.

The **etiology** of post-instrumental pain is usually **multifactorial**. There is no doubt that pain will persist as a result of incomplete instrumentation, e.g., incomplete removal of necrotic and infiltrated pulpal tissues as a result of insufficient debridement or failure to detect secondary root canals. This permits bacteria or their breakdown products (endotoxins) to release pain mediators. In addition, medicinal dressings can have a directly toxic effect or an indirect effect via suppression of host-specific defense mechanisms, leading to postoperative pain. Complete and total removal of all necrotic tissue is the treatment of choice and almost always leads to elimination of pain. Instrumentation of the root canal should always proceed from the coronal toward the apical region, accompanied by copious rinsing with NaOCl.

An additional cause for the appearance of postoperative discomfort is forcing necrotic tissue residues through the apex during canal instrumentation. Despite precise working length determination, if the instruments are improperly used, **extrusion** of debris through the apical foramen can occur; such debris contains not only necrotic tissue residues, but also viable microorganisms and rinsing solutions. This leads directly to periapical inflammation and a foreign body reaction. If the radiographic working length determination is incorrect, massive overinstrumentation may occur, whereby bacteria are introduced into the otherwise bacteria-free periapical tissues and elicit an acute exacerbation extending from the already chronically inflamed periapical lesion.

Debris extrusion occurs after all types of root canal instrumentation, but "balanced-force" rotatory techniques elicit only minimal extrusion, especially after broad coronal opening and subsequent apical instrumentation of the root canal. Conventional hand instrumentation (step-back) leads to the most severe debris extrusion.

There exist varying opinions about the possible role of overfilling the root canal with gutta percha and sealer in terms of occurrence of postoperative discomfort. Torabinejad found in a clinical study **no** relationship between root canal filling length (e.g., overfilling) and the intensity of postoperative pain.

Postoperative discomfort following retreatment of a failed endodontic procedure occurs much more often than following the initial treatment. After a one-visit endodontic treatment, only 2% of patients will exhibit severe pain; however, statistical studies reveal there is no difference between the occurrences of postoperative pain in one-visit or two-appointment endodontic treatment.

It is interesting to note that postoperative pain is especially frequent in apprehensive patients.

Without any doubt, the best method to **prevent** postoperative pain is an effective emergency procedure including complete debridement of the root canal using the **crown-down method** to achieve "apical patency," e.g., a completely patent root canal. The use of a one-week chlorhexidine gel interim dressing reduces bacterial number and the release of toxins.

Case Presentation

A Emergency treatment with incomplete root canal instrumentation and application of Ledermix.

B/C Seven days later, the canals were rinsed and working length was determined with slight overinstrumentation; subsequently, the canal was fully debrided and a calcium hydroxide dressing was placed.

D Twenty-four hours later, the patient presented with significant swelling as a result of the extrusion of necrotic tissue.

E Following intraoral incision and release of suppuration, the patient's pain symptoms immediately subsided.

F–H Five days after reduction of the acute symptoms, the canal was again instrumented, and definitively filled two months later.

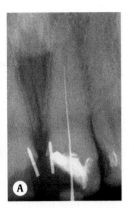

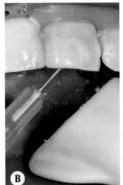

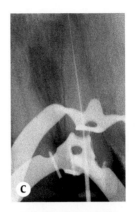

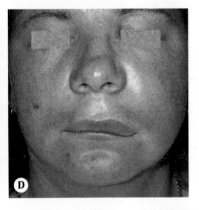

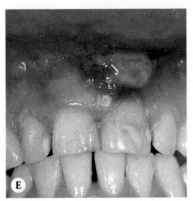

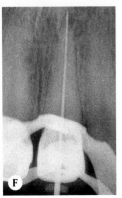

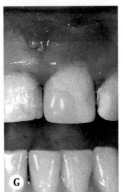

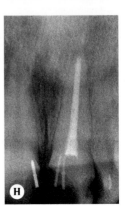

The **diagnosis** of acute periapical lesions is arrived at via clinical examination and through interpretation of the radiograph. The tooth is pressure and percussion sensitive and usually mobile, as well as slightly extruded from its alveolus. Quite often one also notes swelling of the adjacent soft tissue. With acute periapical inflammation, fistula formation is unlikely. However, a fistula may close spontaneously, and in this phase acute symptoms will occur. The swelling may be fluctuant, localized or diffuse, and may occur intraorally and/or extraorally.

The **goal of treatment** is achieving efficient **drainage** with **efflux of pus**; all further steps of treatment are analogous to the treatment for a necrotic pulp.

If the soft tissue **swelling** is **localized**, the affected tooth should be opened to permit drainage via the root canal. In most patients, the coronal aspect is initially expanded and this accomplishes removal of most of the infected tissue. Subsequently, a #15 Hedström file is used to reach the root apex and slightly widen the root canal. The tooth should be stabilized, and the rubber dam clamp applied only on adjacent teeth. In many patients, pus escapes immediately upon trepanation, but only in a few patients is it possible to extend the file 0.5–1 mm beyond the apex. If a relatively **large and fluctuant swelling** is present, and if it does not become smaller following release of pus via the root canal, soft tissue incision and drainage may be indicated. In every case, the canals must be initially instrumented, rinsed, filled with CHX gel, and closed coronally.

If there is adequate drainage via the root canal, the tooth is left open for only 20 minutes with the rubber dam in place, the canal is instrumented 1–2 file sizes and then filled with CHX gel and the cavity closed for three to five days with Cavit. Only during the second appointment is the root canal completely instrumented and then treated for four weeks with a Calxyl dressing.

In the case of **diffuse swelling**, there is no indication for incision, rather the patient must be treated systemically with an antibiotic, and the root canal completely instrumented. The canal is alternately rinsed with sodium hypochlorite and 0.2% chlorhexidine, subsequently also with an EDTA-containing solution (e.g., Calcinase) and then again with NaOCl. After thoroughly drying the canal, a mixture of calcium hydroxide and chlorhexidine is rotated gently into the canal, and the patient is appointed 14 hours later.

Leaving the tooth open after trepanation is only indicated for general systemic medical conditions or poor patient cooperation that makes thorough trepanation and instrumentation impossible. In such cases, instrumentation and closure of the tooth should occur no later than six days after the initial appointment. If the root canal remains open beyond this period, additional bacterial colonization will occur, as well as impaction of food debris.

There exist only five **reasons to prescribe antibiotics**: as a prophylactic measure for systemic medical conditions, diffuse swelling, diffuse abscess, lymphadenopathy, fever, as well as evulsion or luxation of the affected tooth. Pain is not an adequate reason for prescribing antibiotics if no sufficient diagnosis has been established. If the patient requires antibiotic coverage, **penicillin and its derivatives** are the treatments of first choice. Erythromycin represents an alternative. The patient must be appointed every second day for control; during the first 24 hours, the swelling may actually increase.

Case Presentation

A A 2-cm, fluctuant swelling is obvious on the palate, emanating from the maxillary first premolar.

B Suppuration via the root canal, which should be left open for about 20 minutes, and then the root canal is completely instrumented.

C During this initial appointment, the infected tissue is removed and Ca(OH)$_2$ is gently rotated in.

D The radiograph exhibits an obvious periapical radiolucency as well as the measurement files in situ.

E Three weeks later, the palatal swelling was no longer apparent.

F Radiographic view of the completed endodontic treatment.

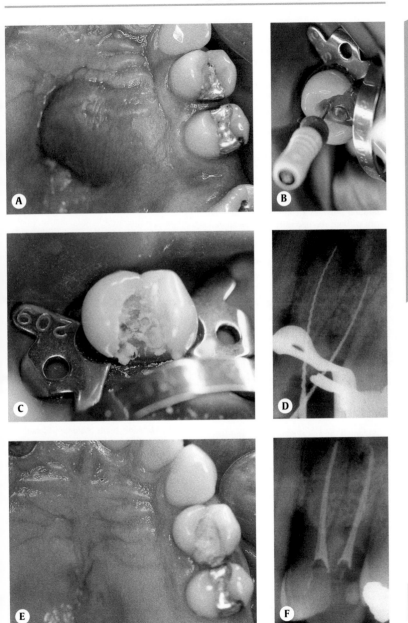

In the great majority of patients, periapical lesions disappear following purely conservative endodontic treatment. One clinical study reported a success rate of 94.5%. The failure rate was 1.8% following vital extirpation and 6.7% for necrotic pulps. Such conservatively attainable success is critically dependent upon effective instrumentation of the root canal, antibacterial rinsing, and a definitive filling that is impervious to bacteria.

With periapical lesions over 20mm in diameter, it is reasonable to assume that in most patients a cyst is present, however neither clinical nor radiographic examination can provide definitive differentiation. With such large periapical lesions, the process of **marsupialization** provides a connection to the oral cavity without the necessity of surgically removing bone that would be necessary for a cystostomy procedure. Marsupialization can be performed by inserting a tube from the vestibular approach.

A "decompression" can also result from opening the periapical lesion via the root canal. Following canal instrumentation using Gates-Glidden drills, a stainless steel tube with a diameter of 1.2mm is cemented into the canal. The patient must then return several times each week for rinsing of the canal, e.g., with 2% NaOCl solution or chlorhexidine. At each appointment, the embedded tube is ultrasonically cleaned. After three to four months the tube can be removed, the exudation appraised, and a temporary dressing placed.

Widening the apical constriction and rinsing the periapical lesion may occasion numerous **dangers**. If the bacterially infected root canal is overinstrumented, in almost all patients the result is a transient bacteremia; the blood picture reveals peptostreptococci and fusobacteria, among others. Forceful rinsing with sodium hypochlorite elicits an additional acute reaction, with pain, swelling and tissue necrosis; it may also necessitate surgical procedures and should therefore not be considered as a routine endodontic procedure.

If apical trepanation is necessary to permit the efflux of pus via the root canal, only slight overinstrumentation using a 15 Hedström or K file is performed, and the precise length verified radiographically. There has to be a trade-off between the loss of the apical constriction and attendant difficulty in determining the working length on the one hand, and the advantage of releasing accumulated pus without an incision.

Aeration, as described by Schröder, is only rarely indicated, and only if all of the previously described emergency measures have not reduced the pain or were otherwise impossible to perform. Aeration is achieved via a small incision at the height of the root tip; the soft tissue is reflected with an elevator and then a small round bur is used to penetrate the bone up to the root tip.

Case Presentation

A A mandibular first molar was pressure and percussion sensitive. The radiograph revealed a small ca. 20-mm diameter periapical radiolucency. Following trepanation of the pulp chamber and careful instrumentation, there was a massive release of pus from the distal root canal.

B After opening the pulp chamber, the working length was determined radiographically. The apical constriction was expanded in order to elicit additional pus release via the root canal; however, this procedure brings with it serious risks.

C The root canal was instrumented. The coronal and middle thirds could be widened using Gates-Glidden drills to a minimum diameter of 1.2mm.

D Within the root canal, a canula or a stainless steel tube is cemented in, and the rest of the cavity is sealed. Using saline solution, the root canal and the periapical lesion can be rinsed every two days via the tube. Weekly, the tube should be removed from the canal and sterilized.

E/F Eight weeks following marsupialization, as well as three months after placement of temporary dressings, the root canal can be definitively filled. Despite measurement of the gutta percha points, a massive overfilling of the canal occurred because of the lack of an apical stop.

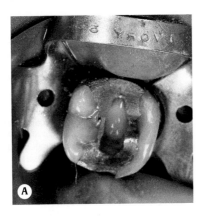

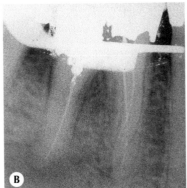

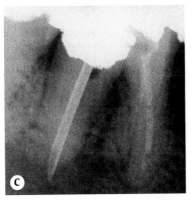

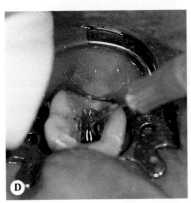

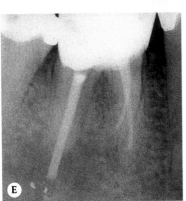

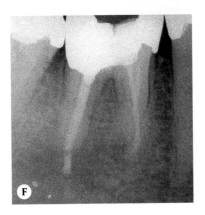

Drainage Not Possible via the Apex

A **periapical abscess** can develop from an **acute apical periodontitis** due to persistence of the bacterial infection within the root canal. Acute apical periodontitis is characterized clinically by percussion sensitivity as well as pain upon axial loading. The periapical abscess may present as an acute lesion or in an encapsulated, chronic form. Initially, the abscess cannot be discerned radiographically. The massive inflammatory cell infiltration in the periapical region and the osteoclastic activity lead to visible bone loss only after three to four weeks.

If the **chronic apical periodontitis** is secondarily infected by bacteria, a **"phoenix abscess"** evolves based on an acute exacerbation of the chronic pathologic process. The radiograph reveals a periapical radiolucency, and clinically one encounters a high degree of percussion sensitivity, tooth elongation, and severe pain. Histologically, the periapical lesion does not exhibit any peculiarities vis-à-vis pain, swelling or fistula formation, in contrast to symptom-free teeth exhibiting apical lesions. Nevertheless, in teeth exhibiting spontaneous pain as well as percussion sensitivity, the root canal exhibits a much more severe bacterial infiltration compared with teeth without clinical symptoms. With percussion, swelling, and exudation, the primary bacterial species are *Streptococcus, Peptostreptococcus, Eubacterium, Porphyromonas,* and *Bacteroides.* The latter are responsible for the typical foul odor emanating from infected root canals.

The persistence of bacterial infection in conjunction with inhibition or reduction of host response can lead to penetration of the suppuration into the surrounding soft tissues, resulting in swelling, fistula formation, or spontaneous pus release; or, it may lead to osteomyelitis. In such cases, **systemic symptoms** such as the swelling of regional lymph nodes and fever occur.

The **treatment** is targeted primarily toward evacuation of the pus. If **drainage** can be established via the root canal, there is no need for incision. Only if root canal drainage cannot be established is **incision** indicated. The armamentarium for incision includes a disposable scalpel, an elevator, as well as an artery clamp. Following successful local anesthesia, an incision is performed at the height of the swelling.

Usually this results in an immediate release of copious amounts of pus. Subsequently, the elevator is used to reflect soft tissue from the bone, and the periosteum is slightly elevated. Thereafter, it may be necessary to insert the closed artery clamp into the abscess cavity and expand the orifice to insure efflux of the suppurative material.

In conjunction with the drainage, rinsing is performed with physiologic saline solution or 3% hydrogen peroxide, and a T-shaped rubber drain is placed into the incision wound. This drain is fabricated from rubber dam material, sterilized, and can be prepared as necessary in various sizes. The drain is then secured with a suture to the surrounding soft tissue and remains for three to five days in the incision opening in order to ensure satisfactory pus evacuation. The patient is reappointed one day later and then also three and five days later; the wound opening is rinsed and the regression of swelling is documented.

After elimination of the acute symptoms, a decision must be made concerning further treatment; this may involve comprehensive endodontic treatment or even extraction of the tooth.

Case Presentation

A This female patient had suffered for one week with increasing pain as well as swelling of the upper lip region extending to the canine fossa.

B The radiograph depicts a periapical radiolucency; the tooth had been trephined one year earlier and left open.

C Tooth 22 is fractured at the level of the gingiva and is extremely percussion sensitive.

D As an emergency procedure, a palatal incision was made. An excision would have been preferable to prevent closure of the mucosal surfaces.

E Following root canal instrumentation during the first appointment, the canal was prepared for a temporary prosthetic replacement and the root canal was securely closed coronally.

F Radiographic view three months after emergency therapy; indication of osseous regeneration.

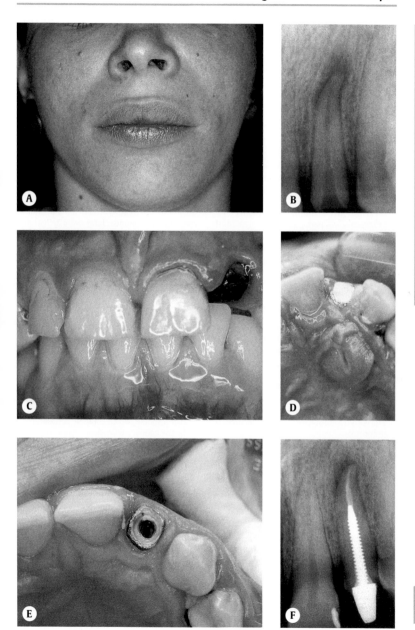

Various studies in the literature report the **prevalence** of radicular cysts between 6–55% of all periapical lesions. In one study, 2308 lesions were submitted by 314 dentists. The specimens were not ideal, consisting of less than comparable surgical preparations that were often of poor quality, providing but few truly evaluable sections. Therefore, the discrepancy in the reported incidence of radicular cysts results from varying interpretation of the various histologic sections. This premise was very well supported by the study of Nair, in which 52% of all periapical lesions exhibited an epithelial lining, but only 15% conformed strictly to the definition of a periapical, radicular cyst. In 35%, the diagnosis of abscess was given, and in an additional 50%, the diagnosis was periapical granuloma. Most significant was the finding that **two classes of radicular cysts** may be encountered:

- true periapical cysts with complete epithelial lining of the cavity
- periapical pocket cysts whose lumen is open to the root canal.

Only 9% of the periapical lesions examined histologically were shown to be **true cysts**. The existence of two classes of radicular cysts, and the low incidence of true cysts determine the decision for surgical removal of these lesions, which are only detected radiographically. Statistics have shown that about every second periapical lesion is treated surgically, and this reveals that a disproportionately large number of surgical procedures are performed at the root tip.

Clinically, one encounters a true radicular cyst in only about 10% of patients; therefore, the majority of periapical lesions can be cured by purely orthograde root canal treatment. Critical, of course, is a correct diagnosis. In a recent study, 43 root tip resection specimens were examined clinically and bacteriologically. Radiographically, in 12 cases radicular cysts were identified, and in 31 cases "noncystic" granulomatous inflammation. The histology revealed 25 instances of chronic inflammation ("granuloma"), for a total of 58.15%, followed by eight abscesses (18.6%) and 10 cysts (23.25%). Chronic and acute inflammatory cells were **always** found together. Only **one** of the cases classified clinically as a cyst could be corroborated by histologic examination. Of the 31 lesions classified as "noncysts" preoperatively, eight exhibited all signs of a "true" cyst; one was classified as a pocket cyst.

In summary, it may be concluded that **no correlation exists between the radiographic diagnosis and the histological findings for the diagnosis of a radicular cyst**.

The clinical consequences of this conclusion are extremely important, indicating that every periapical lesion should be treated **purely conservatively** if this is technically possible. Only during the course of further radiographic examination after conclusion of routine root canal treatment and even the prosthetic (!) treatment can the clinician **at the earliest six months later** draw a clear and unequivocal **indication for surgical treatment**. If the lesion increases in size, it is an indication for surgical removal of the root tip and elimination of the cyst.

Case Presentation

A/B A 54-year-old patient presented with pain that had persisted for several days. The intraoral examination revealed whitish accumulations and mucosal ulceration in the labial vestibule, which could be accounted for by the patient's topical application of aspirin tablets. The radiograph revealed a periapical radiolucency on tooth 12.

C/D Following trepanation and initial instrumentation with a Hedström file, copious suppurative exudate mixed with blood emanated from the root canal.

E Following root canal instrumentation and rinsing, Calxyl was rotated into the canal.

F With persisting pain, tooth 11 was also treated endodontically.

G The periapical lesion on tooth 12 persisted.

H A radiograph, taken two years following root tip resection of tooth 12, exhibits healthy periapical conditions.

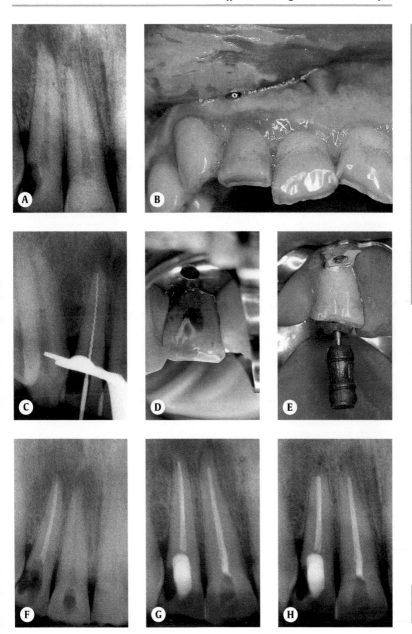

Diverse interconnections between pulpal tissue and the surrounding periodontal tissues can lead to **pathologic interactions**: Pathogenic microorganisms can traverse lateral canals, dentinal tubules, the periodontal ligament, and the alveolar bone, as well as the apical foramina. Most bacterial exchange occurs via the apical foramen, but this is not the only source of communication between the periodontium and the endodontium. Accessory canals in the apical region, as well as in the furcation of molars, provide conduits between both tissues. Inflammation in the interradicular periodontal tissues may be elicited by pulpal inflammation. In 28.4% of molars, there exist such communications in the furcation region, and 10.2% of molars examined exhibited lateral canals further apically.

An **endodontic infection** can lead to expansive alveolar bone resorption and can also modify an existing marginal periodontitis by enhancing periodontal pocket formation through the release of lytic pathogens via lateral canals. It is also possible that irritation of the lateral periodontal tissues may be elicited by medicaments placed into the root canal. A successful (surgical) periodontal treatment, however, almost always leads to healing of the marginal defect independent of any pulpal inflammation.

On the other hand, a **marginal (periodontal) inflammation** that extends to the apical foramen can initiate a **retrograde** pulpitis. Controversy persists regarding whether the pulpitis results from infection of lateral canals or via canals in the furcation. Even though up to 40% of the periodontal attachment is lost, Bergenholtz and Lindhe detected no inflammation in 70% of examined pulps. In the remaining 30%, the pulpal tissue exhibited only minimal inflammation or secondary dentin formation adjacent to the destroyed periodontal tissues. External resorptions were always observed, which made possible the transmission of pathogens via exposed dentinal tubuli. This finding demonstrates the significance of an intact cementum layer on the root surface, which may block the infusion of toxins into the pulpal tissue. Consequently, the existence of pulpitis is highly unlikely to be elicited by marginal periodontitis.

If a primary periodontal lesion with a secondarily elicited pulpitis occurs, and if the patient reports intermittently occurring pain and clinical symptoms of pulpitis, the clinician must consider the possibility of a marginal inflammation extending to the apical foramen. Radiographically, these lesions are difficult to differentiate from a primary endodontic inflammation with secondarily elicited periodontal inflammation. In such cases, both periodontal therapy as well as root canal treatment should be performed.

Root amputation is therefore one of the various treatment methods to prolong the functional life of a tooth that exhibits furcation involvement. The goal is to slow down the process of attachment loss on the remaining root. The rate of loss on remaining roots is only 30% over the long term. After five years, 83% of root-amputated teeth remain, and 68% after 10 years.

Endodontic treatment should be performed **before** periodontal surgical therapy. An exception to this general rule is an indication for hemisection or root amputation discovered during a periodontal flap procedure. If it comes to root amputation, a decision must be made concerning whether the entire tooth crown should be maintained or if some portion of the crown must also be sacrificed. The latter technique affords not only technical advantages but is also more favorable in terms of periodontal prophylaxis, especially when the remaining tooth segment will be used as a bridge abutment.

Case Presentation

A/B Endodontic pretreatment of maxillary second molar exhibiting pronounced bone resorption on both buccal roots.

C Following hemisection and extraction of both buccal roots, plaque accumulation and calculus formation is obvious apically.

D/E Situation six months after removal of the buccal roots and prosthetic treatment using a bridge construction from the palatal root to the canine.

F Initial situation: panoramic radiograph.

G Final result, two years after initiation of treatment.

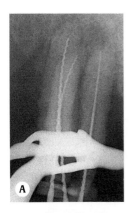

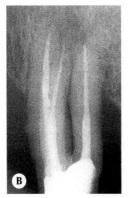

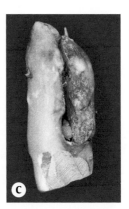

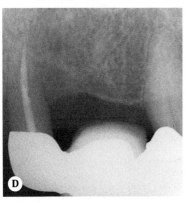

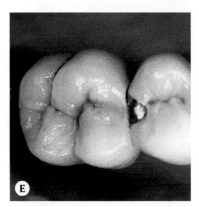

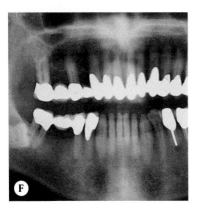

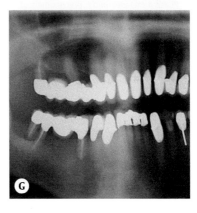

Systematic treatment planning remains, even today, an all too often insufficiently attained goal in daily dental practice. The treatment goal "maintenance of oral structures" demands a comprehensive treatment plan in which all dental disciplines are integrated and temporally sequenced.

To provide a comprehensive overview, treatment planning can be categorized into six typical phases, described below:

The goal of **phase 1** is the formulation of an initial treatment plan with radiographic and periodontal examinations as well as diagnosis and prognosis, *following* elimination of the patient's pain. Treatment planning at this stage can only be preliminary and is related especially to treatment needs, differential therapy, and prognosis of the various treatment methods. Following phase 1, the dentist has a prepared and completely informed patient who is capable of participating in decisions concerning further treatment.

The goal of **phase 2** is **maintenance** of all remaining teeth by means of oral surgical procedures, interim treatment and restorative therapy, endodontic procedures, periodontal treatment, functional therapy, and finally a comprehensive re-evaluation. All clinical findings are recorded during a second data collection appointment.

In **phase 3**, periodontal and endodontic **surgical** procedures are performed. The re-evaluation at the end of this phase permits definitive conclusions concerning which of the initially questionable teeth can be maintained.

Phase 4 includes initial pretreatment procedures for dental implants and/or orthodontic treatment, before any definitive prosthetic therapy (**phase 5**). **Phase 6** may be characterized as the maintenance phase, to secure treatment success over the long term. The definitive treatment plan should include only those teeth that are functionally and aesthetically significant, and possess an adequately positive prognosis. Endodontic treatment can be performed in virtually all patients.

Indications for endodontic treatment include an irreversibly damaged or necrotic pulp with or without clinical or radiographic evidence of periapical involvement. Questionable pulpal condition in the face of anticipated restorative therapy is an important indication.

Contraindications include teeth that cannot be functionally restored as well as those with an unfavorable periodontal prognosis, and a poor overall oral health condition.

Indications for retreatment include teeth with inadequate root canal filling, with pathologic radiographic findings, and/or clinical symptoms, as well as when the coronal restoration needs to the replaced. A recent study demonstrated that 60% of all endodontically treated teeth exhibit an apical radiolucency as an indication of treatment failure. This relates first to improper case selection and second to the treatment technique employed. Any postendodontic pathology necessitates intervention, which can be performed orthograde or retrograde. **Orthograde revision** is preferred based on its advantages and the low risk in contrast to apical surgery. Each case must be carefully considered to determine if retreatment is even possible. The success rate following retreatment is about 70%, which is clearly below that for initial endodontic treatment. A decision to attempt retreatment must also take into consideration the higher levels of technical skills and time commitment required.

Case Presentation

A The radiograph of tooth 25 reveals an inadequate root canal filling and an obvious periapical radiolucency. Tooth 24 exhibits no root canal filling, rather only a short post build-up.

B After removing the bridge from 13 to 23/24, the build-up on tooth 24 was obvious.

C After dissolution with eucalyptol, the gutta percha was removed from tooth 25 and two canals were reinstrumented.

D Radiograph of the retreated root canal; orthograde radiographic projection.

E Using an excentric radiographic projection, both premolars exhibit a second canal, which was likely the etiology of the periapical radiolucency on tooth 25.

F Clinical view after seating the new bridge.

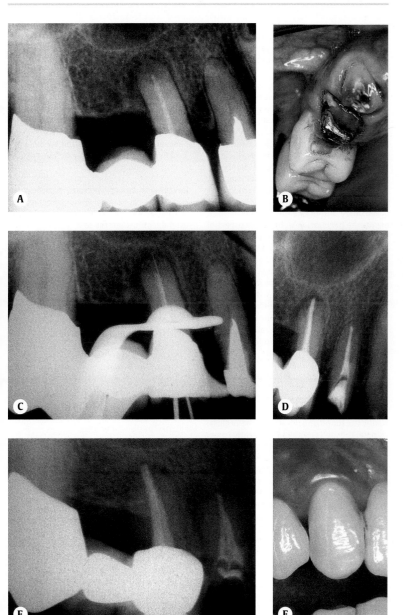

Local Anesthesia

Treatment Planning and Preparation

It is important to inject **slowly**. Rapid injection of even small amounts of solution cause considerable pressure within the soft tissue; this can elicit pain, which is more severe with dense connective tissue.

It is absolutely necessary to **aspirate** twice. Inadvertent intravascular injection can lead to toxic reactions. The risk is highest with nerve block anesthesia. Administration of block anesthesia at the mandibular foramen will involve vascular puncture in 11% of patients. In 2% of all intraoral injections, blood will be aspirated. Following the first aspiration, the syringe is rotated 90° or 180° along its long axis. In **half** of all patients, blood appears in the carpule following the second aspiration.

Maxillary anterior teeth are anesthetized via needle penetration in the labile aspect of the vestibular fold, with the needle parallel to the tooth's long axis and deposition of ca. 1 ml of solution. Immediately after penetrating the mucosa, a few drops of solution are injected before inserting the needle to its final position. For **maxillary posterior teeth**, the needle is inserted mesial to the affected tooth and positioned superiorly-posteriorly over the root tip. Block anesthesia of the anterior palatal nerve is only necessary for **surgical** endodontic procedures.

Anesthesia in the mandible is achieved by blocking the trunk or branches of the inferior alveolar nerve in the pterygomandibular space immediately before entry of the nerve into the mandibular foramen. In 22.5% of patients, the foramen is located at the occlusal plane of the molars, and in 75% slightly below that plane. Some authors have also reported foramina in the retromolar fossa, which provide ingress for accessory nerve fibers to the mandibular molars. In three out of eight patients, direct connections exist between these nerves and branches of the inferior alveolar nerve. Thus, to achieve profound anesthesia of mandibular molars, it is prudent to inject less solution in the retromolar region. In addition, the mylohyoid nerve may play some role in the innervation of mandibular posterior teeth. In 53% of patients, accessory foramina exist in the mylohyoid fovea, which contain pain and temperature fibers. Other authors have described accessory foramina on the lingual aspect of the posterior mandibular region.

Complications with nerve block anesthesia at the mandibular foramen include:
- A temporary paresthesia of the ipsilateral facial muscle due to anesthesia of the facial nerve resulting from deposition of anaesthetic solution too far posteriorly.
- Blockade of the stellate ganglion caused by the influx of anaesthetic solution through the pharyngeal space and paravertebrally. The result is a flushing of the ipsilateral side of the face, ptosis of the eyelid, and a rash in the neck region extending to the arm on the same side.

Direct nerve damage will cause persistent anesthesia or paresthesia. During the injection, the patient will report an "electric jolt," which extends throughout the region served by that nerve.

Anesthesia in Various Intraoral Areas

A The target for the inferior alveolar nerve is within the pterygomandibular space immediately before its entrance into the mandibular canal. The foramen is at the height of the molar occlusal surfaces. The needle is inserted parallel to the occlusal surface until contact with bone, somewhat superior to the lingula. At least 1.5 ml of anaesthetic solution is then slowly injected.

B In the maxillary posterior region, the anaesthetic solution is deposited posterior to the maxillary alveolar process.

C *Endodontic surgical procedures in the maxillary anterior segment:* Initiate the injection vestibularly near tooth 21, and subsequently palatal to the nasopalatine nerve.

D *Posterior segment:* Initiate the injection vestibularly from tooth 27, then palatally. Right: injection for operation on the palatal root of tooth 16.

E *Mandibular posterior tooth region:* The injection is initiated with block anesthesia at the mandibular canal, subsequently in the vestibule, and then lingual to tooth 47.

F *Anterior mandible:* Initially, block anesthesia at the mandibular canal, then within the vestibule, and also lingually.

80

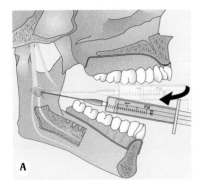

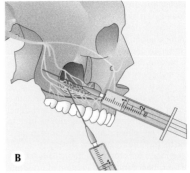

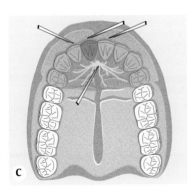

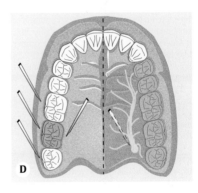

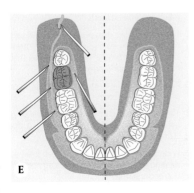

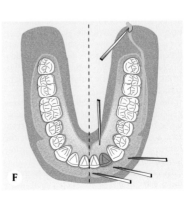

Endodontic treatment should **only** be performed on a tooth that has been isolated with the rubber dam, in order to avoid bacterial contamination and influx of saliva, to prevent aspiration or swallowing of instruments and to prevent the escape of rinsing solutions into the oral cavity. Generally speaking, if a tooth is so broken down that a rubber dam cannot be effectively placed, extraction may represent a better therapeutic alternative. In exceptional cases, the adjacent teeth may also be used to receive the rubber dam clamp, for example if the tooth to be treated has already been prepared for a full crown. Additional **advantages of the rubber dam** are, in addition to an aseptic working field, retraction of the soft tissue, significantly better vision and easier access for the endodontic instruments, time saving, and generally improved quality as experienced by the patient. Nevertheless, the acceptance of rubber dam isolation varies considerably: 50% of American dentists regularly use the rubber dam for endodontic treatment, but only 20% of Swiss dentists and only 8% of German dentists.

The rubber dam as a system for maintaining a dry operating field was proposed in 1864 by S.C. Barnum. In 1870, the first clamps appeared on the market, and in 1943, latex replaced India rubber.

The rubber dam armamentarium consists of the latex rubber, a frame, rubber dam punch and application forceps, as well as rubber dam clamps and various aids such as dental floss, and the rubber dam napkin.

The **rubber dam material** is available as heavy, extra heavy, or medium strength. Precut sheets (15×15 cm) are available, and for patients with latex allergy, nonlatex rubber is available. However, the latter is more difficult to apply and tears easily; in addition, it is susceptible to dissolution when eucalyptol is used during retreatment of gutta percha root canal fillings.

The rubber dam is stretched onto a **frame** made of metal (Young) or plastic. Traditional plastic rubber dam frames are available from Osty, a radiolucent frame from Hygenic, the Visiframe from Starlite and the collapsible frame from Sauveur.

The **rubber dam punch** is used to create round perforations in the rubber dam material. Two types of punches (Ivory, Ainsworth) are differentiated by the position of the hinge. Both types have a round plate with five or six holes of various sizes (0.5–2 mm). The tip of the punch penetrates the rubber dam, creating a hole that is appropriate for the affected tooth.

Rubber dam pliers are used to expand the clamp in order to position it on the tooth. There are three different types: In type 1, the arms are straight except for a sharp bend at the end; in type 2, the arms exhibit several bends; with type 3, the clamps can only be used on one side.

Rubber dam clamps are available with or without wings (W). Clamps are available for distal (D), anterior tooth, premolars, and molars for retention or retraction. Among the numerous types of clamps, sets consisting of four to eight clamps are recommended, e.g., #212 for anterior teeth, #0, 1, and 2 for premolars, #7, 8, 8A, and 14A for molars.

Rubber Dam Application

A Latex rubber (15×15 cm), medium strength, in blue or green color for good contrast, is stretched upon an appropriate plastic or metal frame. A special soft-cloth barrier is placed between the skin and the rubber dam. Foldable frames made of plastic have the advantauge that they do not have to be removed during radiography, but are often cumbersome to use.

B Clamps for molars: above, #7 with straight beaks and below #8A for severely broken-down or prepared teeth.

C The Ivory rubber dam punch (left) produces reliably good holes that do not tear; at right is the punch from Ainsworth, a model that has remained unchanged for 100 years!

D Punch plate of the Ivory device with six holes of 1–2 mm diameter.

E The Ivory rubber dam pliers have a steel sling behind the hinge that permits holding the clamp in its open position.

F Wide stops at the tip of each beak prevent slipping or excessively deep (apical) application of the clamp.

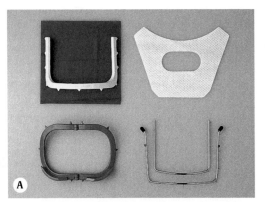

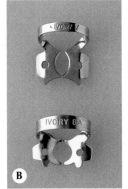

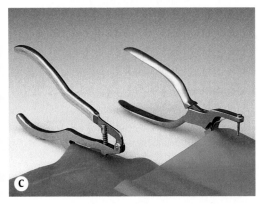

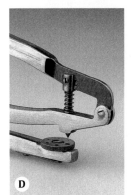

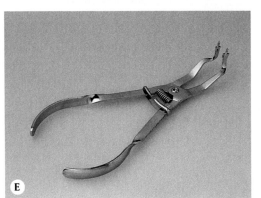

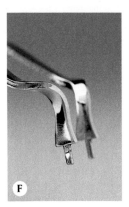

Many considerations go into each rubber dam application: informing the patient about materials and procedures, consideration of the clinical situation (e.g., remaining tooth crown), selection of rubber dam material and clamps, as well as the location and size of the perforations in the rubber dam material.

Applying the rubber dam can be done in four different ways. For endodontics, the most reasonable approach is **simultaneous application of the clamp and the rubber dam**. In this so-called **wing technique**, there are two phases: preparation by the dental assistant and the actual application in the patient's mouth. After punching an appropriately sized hole in the rubber dam, both wings of the clamp are inserted below the rubber. Thereafter, the rubber dam is stretched onto the frame. When this combination of clamp, rubber dam pliers, rubber dam material, and frame is mounted, the time at chairside is reduced to a minimum. Careful application of the clamp apical to the height of contour of the tooth must be determined with the patient's participation to prevent any encroachment or damage to the gingiva. Application is completed with the reflection of the stretched rubber over the clamp wings using a Heidemann spatula and adapting the rubber into the proximal spaces using dental floss.

Using the **bow technique**, the index finger is used to position the rubber over the rubber dam pliers at the height of the hinge. The dam is then stretched over the wings of the clamp using the other hand, and folded anteriorly. Then the clamp is positioned on the tooth and the rubber is stretched over the wings and around the tooth. The frame is then positioned and attached.

In the third method, the punched rubber is first stretched over the tooth and the clamp is then placed. This technique is always used with the #212 clamp on **anterior teeth**.

For other applications, the **clamp** can be **adjusted on the tooth** initially. For this technique, wingless clamps are usually employed, which permit and simplify stretching the rubber dam into place. The rubber is severely stretched over the distal arch of the clamp. Then it is stretched over the buccal and the lingual aspects of the clamp, and attached to the frame.

In certain clinical situations it may be necessary to modify the dam application technique in order to isolate the tooth fully. Aids in this regard include dental floss, Wedjets, Kerr compound, or Cavit.

Single-tooth isolation, which is preferred for endodontic treatment, may need to be enhanced in rare cases using **multitooth isolation**. Depending upon the number of teeth to be isolated, the rubber dam is punched according to a standard **template**. Using the wing technique, the first tooth is isolated and then the rubber is stretched over the additional teeth. Simultaneously, the dental assistant uses dental floss to tease the rubber dam into the interdental spaces. A clamp is also positioned on the most distal tooth and its firm positioning checked using dental floss.

In rare cases, a severely broken-down tooth must be built up before rubber dam application, or a clamp with apically directed beaks must be used subgingivally. Because this technique often elicits gingival trauma, the method must be reserved for exceptional cases.

Case Presentation

A The clamp wings are positioned beneath the rubber and the dam is loosely attached to a frame.

B The rubber dam pliers is inserted into the clamp, and the combination of rubber dam, frame, pliers and clamp are carried to the oral cavity and positioned on the tooth; tension on the clamp is released, the clamp is definitively positioned on the tooth and the pliers are removed.

C The clamp is positioned on tooth 36 and the pliers have been removed.

D/E Using a Heidemann spatula, the rubber is stretched over the wings of the clamp.

E Using dental floss, the rubber is positioned into and below the contact point of the proximal tooth surfaces; the dental floss is removed from the lateral approach.

G/H Rubber dam in its definitive position. The cloth napkin is visible beneath the rubber dam.

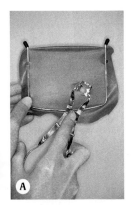

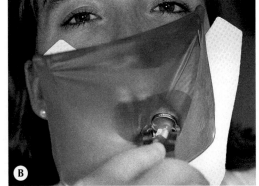

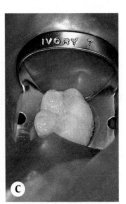

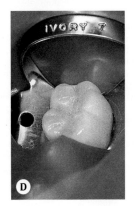

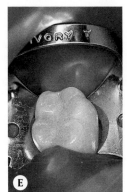

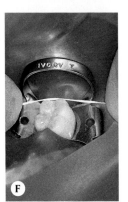

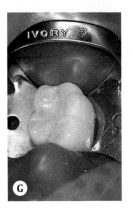

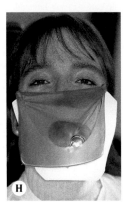

Endodontic treatment begins with the **trepanation**, which is performed with the rubber dam in place. Difficulties during instrumentation of the root canal occur most often as the result of inadequate trepanation and the lack of a **straight-line access** to the root canals. The entrance to the root canal must provide **direct vision**, and this may also require the use of magnifying **loupes** or a surgical microscope.

Coronal hard substance must however be maintained as much as possible; enamel and dentin should only be removed as absolutely necessary. Nevertheless, an excessively small trepanation opening must not inhibit the detection and localization of the root canal orifices. Errors in the creation of the trepanation opening occasion a host of difficulties during the entire endodontic treatment procedure.

The lack of a direct, straight-line access to the root canal orifices may result in straightening of a dilacerated root canal, or even a highly unfavorable perforation. The shape and form of the trepanation opening depends upon complete knowledge of tooth and root canal anatomy because the coronal opening provides an enlarged view of the pulp chamber.

Endodontic therapy presupposes complete removal of all carious substance as well as inadequate restorations. This precludes penetration and consequent contamination of the root canal by bacteria, which would lead to endodontic failure over the long term. Bacteria invade and penetrate dentinal tubuli, colonize there, proliferate relatively uninhibited, and can occasion later periapical inflammation and osseous destruction.

If old restorations are not completely removed, particles of restorative material could be released during instrumentation and block the root canal. If old restorations are intact and do not exhibit any discrepancies radiographically, they may be left intact. On the other hand, however, only after complete removal of restorations or crowns can the extent of carious penetration as well as inadequate areas be established and the root canal orifices better revealed.

In many cases, it is necessary to fabricate a temporary crown or an adhesive restoration to seal the tooth and to protect against fracture during the endodontic treatment.

One problem during trepanation of the pulp cavity is incorrect estimation of the angle between the crown and the root. This makes it more difficult to locate the canal entrances. The diagnostic **radiograph** is extremely helpful for precise localization of the root canal orifices. With extensive coronal restorations, a bitewing radiograph should also be taken. In order to prevent perforation or excessive instrumentation at the cavity floor, the length of the diamond bur should be oriented vis-à-vis the radiograph.

Spherical diamond burs are used initially to achieve the appropriate depth, and cylindrical burs are used to remove hard structure laterally. The **Endo-Access bur** provides a useful combination for the entire trepanation procedure (H. Martin; Maillefer, Ballaigues, Switzerland).

If the canal orifices are undetectable, the dentist should orient toward the largest root canal. The floor of the coronal pulp provides hints about the number and position of canal orifices via color differences, discrete ledges, and grooves revealing the number and position of canal orifices; the roof must, however, be completely removed. It may be prudent to **stain** the floor of the pulpal chamber.

Case Presentation

A Maxillary first molar with an inadequate composite restoration; the radiograph also revealed an inadequate root canal filling.

B After removal of the composite restoration, expansive secondary caries was obvious.

C With direct vision, the caries and infected hard tissues were completely removed and the entrances to the root canals were revealed.

D Clinical view following coronal cavity expansion and instrumentation of all four root canals.

E The root canals were instrumented initially coronally and the working length was determined radiographically.

F Radiographic view of the completed endodontic treatment.

G Radiograph taken four years later.

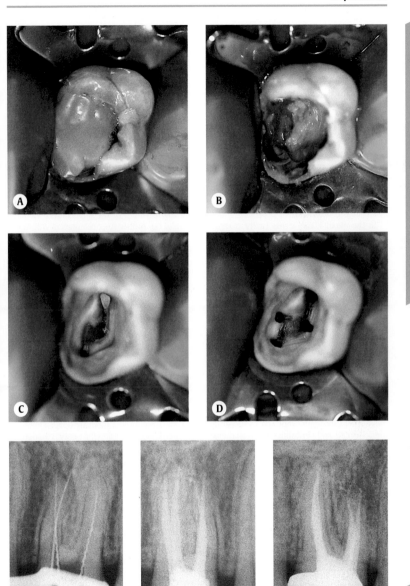

The outline form of an endodontic access cavity corresponds to the shape of the pulp chamber. In **anterior teeth**, access is via a lingual approach. The shape of the cavity in maxillary incisors is triangular, in the center of the palatal surface. It must be sufficiently extended mesially and distally so that the pulp horns can be completely accessed and all necrotic tissue removed. Tissues that are left behind can lead later on to discoloration of the clinical crown. The pulp chamber is prepared at a 45° angle to the long axis of the tooth.

The shape of the access cavity for **mandibular molars** is trapezoidal. The initial trepanation is performed centrally with the axis of the bur distally because the space above the distal canal is easiest to localize.

In the maxilla, the access cavity is rhomboid in shape. The initial trepanation begins in the center of the occlusal surface, tilting the bur toward the mesiopalatal cusp, because the pulp chamber is most expansive here. Once the pulp chamber is encountered, the bur is moved buccally in contact with the pulpal floor in order to remove any overhanging enamel.

Following the initial penetration through the pulp chamber roof above the palatal canal entrance, the extension is completed. In the maxilla, the position of the palatal root canal in molars helps to locate the other canal orifices.

The diamond bur, in contact with the floor of the pulp chamber, is moved buccally to remove the overhanging roof and to reveal the mesiobuccal and distobuccal canals. Final preparation is performed using a diamond bur with a smooth tip. The walls of the access cavity diverge coronally.

The final form of the cavity provides unimpeded access to all root canals. This permits straight and direct access for the root canal instruments. Because many root canals are bent near the coronal segment, all cervical ledges as well as the coronal curvature must be carefully removed. If one encounters difficulty later in the pulp chamber, a slow-speed **Access Bur** (size #1) is used in the dry cavity in the direction of the anticipated canal orifices to a depth of 2 mm.

The floor of the pulp chamber is usually 1–2 mm apical to the cementoenamel junction. If localization of the pulp chamber is difficult, the **distance** can be measured on the **radiograph** and transferred to the Endo-Access bur. A **periodontal probe** can also be helpful for such measurements, to prevent perforations. Maxillary first molars usually have three roots with four root canals; the mesiobuccal root contains the fourth canal. Both mesial canals may overlap when viewed on a buccopalatal radiograph. The use of a second, excentric projection often provides better differentiation.

An additional complication is apical dilaceration distally and palatally. Using a prebent instrument, the course and direction must be tactilely ascertained before instrumentation. The adjustable stop reveals the canal's course in the direction of the dilaceration. Without use of the rubber stop, orientation within the root canal is impossible.

Illustrations

A Note the dentin overhangs, which render difficult any straight-line access, and which therefore increase the danger of instrument breakage.

B Trepanation is performed with an Endo-Access bur, which extends to the appropriate depth and is then used to create the access cavity with diverging walls.

C The prepared cavity access makes possible unimpeded access for instrumentation.

D Maxillary anterior teeth are opened from the palatal approach and the cavity is triangular.

E Maxillary premolars are opened with an oval profile in the orovestibular direction.

F Maxillary molars are opened with a rhomboid or trapezoidal access.

G Mandibular incisors and canines will exhibit two root canals in 25% of patients, and the access approach is from the lingual.

H Trepanation of premolars is an oval approach in the orovestibular direction, from the occlusal.

I Molars are opened with a trapezoidal shape, usually somewhat wider at the mesial aspect, but maintaining the mesial marginal ridge.

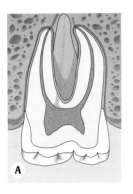

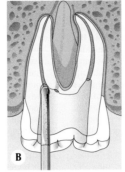

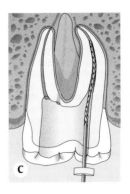

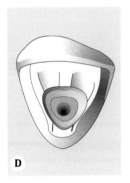

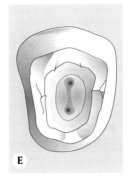

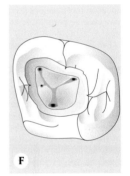

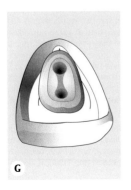

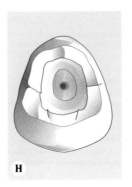

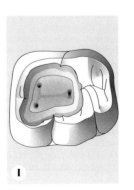

The primary cause of endodontic failure is overlooked root canals. About 40% of all mandibular incisors have two root canals, but only in 1% are there separate apical foramina. Before initiating trepanation, both orthoradial and excentric radiographic projections must be made in order to better demonstrate any anatomic variations. **Maxillary first premolars** will exhibit an additional root canal in ca. 84% of patients; this figure is 58% for second premolars. In addition, 8% of first premolars will exhibit three or more primary ramifications.

During embryologic development, the mesiobuccal and palatal roots of the **maxillary first molar** share a single primary root canal. During tooth development, some cellular segments invaginate and there is deposition of hard tissue; the palatal segment in the mesiobuccal root develops less prominently, and may even be partially or completely obliterated.

Endodontic failures in maxillary molars often result from insufficient instrumentation or completely untreated canals and foramina.

For example, the presence for a fourth root canal in maxillary first molars varies between 19–77% depending upon the method of investigation, and between 10–38% in maxillary second molars. Recent studies have even demonstrated that in 90% of first molars and 70% of second maxillary molars there are two root canals in the mesiobuccal root; therefore, **most** of these teeth will have four root canals. In 52.4% there were two separate canals that converged immediately before the apex; 33% had two separate canals and in 4.8% there was a canal that branched into two separate canals at the apical region.

A solid understanding of the tooth anatomy that may be encountered following trepanation, including the number and the course of the various root canals, represents the basis for successful endodontic therapy. For a better and more comprehensive understanding of the myriad of anatomical variations, various **classifications** have been proposed. In the very comprehensive classification by Vertucci, the **number of canals** is differentiated into those that (1) begin at the floor of the pulp chamber; (2) emerge throughout the course of the canal; and (3) open at the apical foramen.

This classification describes eight types of **canal configurations**:
1. one single canal
2. two confluent canals
3. one branching canal
4. two separate canals
5. one canal that branches immediately before the foramen
6. two canals that unite within the root
7. one canal that branches, reunites and branches again
8. three separate canals within a single root.

Clearly, root canal anatomy cannot always be predicted, and this can be the source of failure. In order to eliminate this possibility, an adequately large trepanation opening that provides good visual access must be made, as well as conventional radiographs and those taken with excentric central ray projection. A special situation is the C-shaped canal. The diagnosis is difficult. Clinical clues include constant and persisting pain, persistent bleeding from the canal as well as confluent lumina following trepanation. The radiographic appearance of the roots is often conical or fused.

Illustrations

A The maxillary first premolar usually presents canal types 4–7, e.g., with two canals that are either completely separate, or which course more or less together. In mandibular premolars, 70% exhibit type 1 with a single root canal. Only with first premolars does one encounter configurations 4 or 5 in 25% of cases.

B The mandibular first molar has two roots: The mesial root has two canals that in 40–45% of cases terminate at a common apical foramen. In the diagram, the distal root is sectioned in the orovestibular plane and exhibits essentially a single root canal. In 27% of cases, the first molar has two canals, 14% of which exhibit separate apical foramina; this is a possible cause for persistence of pain.

C Maxillary first molars usually have four root canals. Depending upon the study, in up to 40% the mesiobuccal root exhibits two separately coursing canals (mesiobuccal, mesiopalatal).

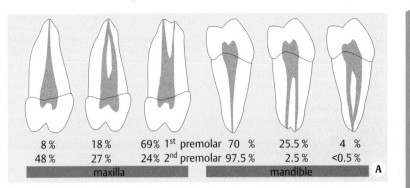

8 %	18 %	69%	1st premolar	70 %	25.5 %	4 %
48 %	27 %	24%	2nd premolar	97.5 %	2.5 %	<0.5 %
maxilla				mandible			**A**

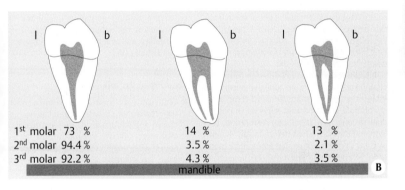

l	b	l	b	l	b
1st molar 73 %		14 %		13 %	
2nd molar 94.4 %		3.5 %		2.1 %	
3rd molar 92.2 %		4.3 %		3.5 %	
mandible						**B**

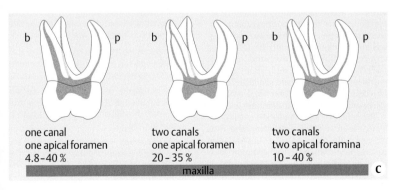

one canal
one apical foramen
4.8–40 %

two canals
one apical foramen
20–35 %

two canals
two apical foramina
10–40 %

maxilla **C**

During treatment planning, only teeth with a **favorable prognosis** should be included, those that are amendable to prosthetic reconstruction. After removal of old restorations, it is necessary to fabricate a temporary that will provide a coronally reproducible **reference point** for determining endodontic working length, and to protect the tooth between appointments from overloading or fracture. In addition, an **impervious closure** against the oral milieu is necessary to prevent salivary ingress and bacterial contamination. Invitro studies have demonstrated that insufficient coronal closure leads to severe microbial re-infection of the root canal after only seven days.

While the endodontic access cavity preparation weakens the tooth by only about 5%, an additional MOD cavity preparation reduces the mechanical strength by about 63%. This clinical fact increases the danger of tooth fracture between appointments. Given this fact, it is prudent to provide an adhesive restoration or a long-term temporary even before endodontic treatment is initiated.

Interim restoration may take the form of a composite resin filling, an adhesive composite inlay, or a cemented acrylic resin temporary restoration; the latter may serve as an immediate or long-term temporary restoration. The extent of the hard tissue defect and the length of time that the temporary restoration must serve will determine the nature of the interim restoration. Glass ionomer cements, including silver particle reinforced and also light hardened, provide an excellent initial marginal adaptation. Rapidly, though, routine occlusal function leads to a significant loss of substance occlusally and a deterioration of marginal adaptation. For average size posterior tooth composite restorations, a conservative tooth preparation in conjunction with the hardening technique will lead to excellent long-term marginal adaptation. The restorations inserted into box-shaped cavities and bonded using the two-layer technique exhibit ideal marginal values of up to 74% after masticatory loading.

The inherent and rapidly developing polymerization shrinkage of **composite resin** must be compensated by means of a time-consuming insertion and polymerization technique. **Immediate temporaries** can be prepared directly in the patient's mouth or indirectly via an impression of the prepared tooth on a dental stone model. Prefabricated crowns, as well as vacuum-formed splints, can be relined with a useful life of one to three months. A **long-term temporary restoration** with a lifespan of up to six months is the prefabricated, thin-walled crown. Temporary restorations incorporating a reduced metal framework and acrylic resin modeling can be cemented for six months to two years; however, such temporary restorations require additional laboratory work and are relatively expensive.

Within a total case rehabilitation, the use of long-term temporaries is often necessary. The dental technical and clinical preparation of a long-term temporary restoration is expensive; patients may view this as excessive since their only real desire was treatment of a nonvital tooth by means of endodontic therapy. A six-month waiting period before definitive restoration is not supported by scientific or clinical data, and is actually associated with a higher failure rate.

Case Presentation

A Teeth 24 and 25 exhibit inadequate amalgam restorations; tooth fracture has also occurred and this makes subsequent restoration more difficult. The tooth must be restored with an adhesive temporary restoration. This will make it possible to apply the rubber dam and establish a reproducible working length.

B In the diagnostic radiograph, one can observe the coronal destruction of tooth 25.

C Following adhesive seating of the temporary that was fabricated in the laboratory, no contamination of the root canal should occur.

D Temporary, short-term closure of the trepanation opening between two appointments using eugenol-free cement.

E The composite resin build-up can be trephined and the root canal can be instrumented; in addition, the working length is reproducible.

F The radiograph exhibits an easily verified and reproducible coronal reference point; the gutta percha master point can be measured without difficulty.

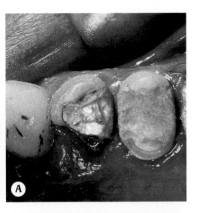

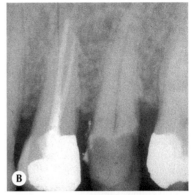

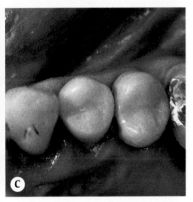

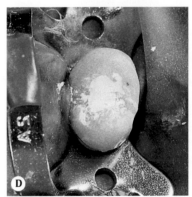

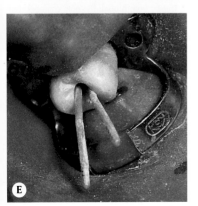

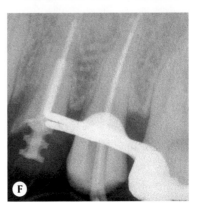

Following penetration of the pulp chamber roof and preparation of the **access cavity**, the root canal orifices are probed. Problems may occur following inadequate removal of the pulp chamber roof. Overhanging dentin must be removed and the cavity must be widened conically toward the occlusal surface. An explorer should be used to determine whether an appropriate amount of dentin has been removed. Visual examination, enhanced by 6–8× magnifying **loupes** together with the use of a front surface **mirror** (HR front, Röder, Ismaning) will determine whether unimpeded access to the canals has been accomplished. Only with optimal illumination and use of magnifying loupes can the details of the floor of the cavity be clearly examined. In many cases, shortening the crown of the tooth will provide an improved visual field.

If the entire coronal cavity is obliterated, the clinician must orient himself according to the color of the dentin. The pulpal floor is gray-brown; the pulpal walls are usually bright and whitish yellow. Calcifications usually exhibit a speckled yellow-brown coloration. These must be removed using a rotating instrument. As soon as the darker pulpal floor is exposed, the largest root canal orifices are sought in the marginal regions. Transillumination from the cervical aspect can be helpful.

Using a thin but firm **probe** (DG 16, Maillefer; EXDG 16, Hu-Friedy), the canal orifices are probed. If the probe sticks, a #15 Hedström file is used to determine whether a root canal has been identified. Only then can the canal orifice begin to be widened coronally.

If the root canal cannot be located, additional tooth preparation must be performed; the cavity must be rinsed and dried and stained if necessary. If the canal orifices are obliterated, the pulpal floor should be re-examined: Gray-black lines will indicate the direction of the canal entrances. If the probe sticks in a suspected root canal, the canal orifice can be exposed using **ultrasonic** activation.

At this point, one begins localizing the **canal orifices** using the shortest possible instruments. Targeted toward this procedure, some instruments of 16 mm in length have been considerably shortened. Especially recom-

mended is the orifice shaper from the Profile-Set of rotating nickel-titanium files. Recommended hand instruments include those from Deepstar and Farside (Maillefer), whose fabrication is based on the characteristics of a reamer. The length of these instruments has been reduced to 15 or 18 mm, and they are available in sizes 06, 08, 10, as well as 15. Because of the reduced length as well as the specially prepared tip, these instruments are easier to insert into the root canals, in comparison to standard instruments.

Some authors have recommended short-term etching of the pulpal floor for 10 seconds or the application of EDTA, to simplify penetration. In exceptional cases, the diamond-coated Endo-Access bur can be used for follow-up preparation. Obliteration of the root canal usually only extends within the short coronal area; in only very rare cases is the entire canal calcified.

Case Presentation

A The radiograph is used to determine the position of the root canal and its orifice within the pulp chamber.

B With the rubber dam in place, the diamond-coated Endo-Access bur is used to penetrate the crown to the appropriate depth.

C Trepanation to the pulp chamber roof.

D Trepanation through the pulp chamber roof and removal of all residual pulpal tissue.

E Localization of the root canal orifices using the special endodontic probe (DG 16, EXDG 16) by probing the floor of the cavity.

F Both canal orifices have been located. Very little hemorrhage occurred; this fact may complicate canal localization.

G Using a #15 Hedström file, the root canal is expanded coronally toward the apical region; this procedure also removes any necrotic pulpal tissue.

H Following coronal expansion, both canal orifices are definitively localized.

I Final radiograph following root canal filling.

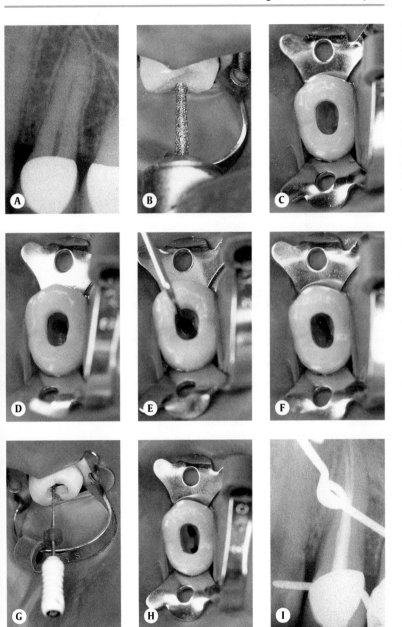

Trepanation and the subsequent probing of the root canal orifices represent the most important measures for endodontic treatment success. The main problems encountered during these procedures include inadequate excavation of caries, leaving behind softened tooth hard substance or inadequate restorations, insufficient access to the pulp chamber, inaccurate estimation of the angle between the crown and the root, inaccurate observation of the tooth within the dental arch, as well as problems during trepanation through the crown, and expansive restorations with consequent obturation of the canal orifice by debris from the fillings.

The complete removal of damaged coronal tooth hard substance must ensure that the remaining enamel/dentin is sufficiently resistant and restorable so that following coronal reconstruction any contamination of the periapical tissues via saliva and bacteria, during endodontic treatment or between appointments, can be prevented. In addition, fracture of the tooth between two appointments must be avoided because this would lead to the loss of a reference point. The excavation of carious tooth structure should always begin at the periphery, leading finally to excavation in the direction of the pulp.

During the process of exposing the root canals, the old adage applies: "Find the pulp horns." However, the pulp horns represent only a small portion of the pulp chamber and reside at the chamber border. Therefore, when the pulp horns are encountered, additional trepanation must be performed and the entire roof of the pulp chamber must be removed in order to expose the canal orifices.

The **radiograph** is used to measure the **depth of the preparation** to the canal orifices, as well as the saggital and transverse dimensions. If the pulp chamber roof is not completely removed, it may not be possible to localize all canal orifices, or it may lead to excessive preparation in an incorrect direction bringing with it the danger of perforation.

If probing of the canal orifices is attended by excessive hemorrhage, rinsing with 5% NaOCl solution should be performed, in extreme cases including 1:50 000 epinephrine on a cotton pellet. Any small **perforations** must be covered with a temporary closure

material such as Cavit, SuperEBA cement, IRM, or with the new MTA cement. In such cases, calcium hydroxide preparations as well as formaldehyde preparations are contraindicated.

A negative result of improper estimation of the angle between crown and root can lead to incorrect assessment of the canals, and failure to detect canals; as a result, tooth hard structure at the pulpal floor may be unnecessarily compromised. If the position of the tooth is far from normal, trepanation should be performed without the rubber dam in place. In exceptional cases, additional crown hard substance must be removed in order to provide adequate visual access to the pulp chamber. During trepanation with the rubber dam in place, a line drawn on the tooth can be used to indicate the crown angle and therewith the direction of trepanation. In some cases it may even be necessary to remove a new prosthetic reconstruction in order to gain adequate visual access.

Case Presentation

A Maxillary first molar after multiple treatment failures; the tooth was left open for two months. The three canals have been well instrumented and completely prepared.

B The radiograph reveals the three roots as well as remnants of the partially removed fillings.

C Following complete removal of the pulp chamber roof, the three canals are clearly visible. Additional preparation was performed ca. 2mm beneath the mesiobuccal canal in the direction of the palatal canal.

D Careful coronal expansion of the canal orifice.

E Radiographic measurement and depiction of the three prepared root canals.

F Careful instrumentation to the working length.

G Detection of the fourth (mesiopalatal) canal and complete coronal expansion of all canals.

H Radiographic view after filling all four root canals. The patient was free of symptoms. The etiology of the previous persistent pain was the infected, separate mesiopalatal root canal.

I Direct view into the cavity following completion of the root canal fillings.

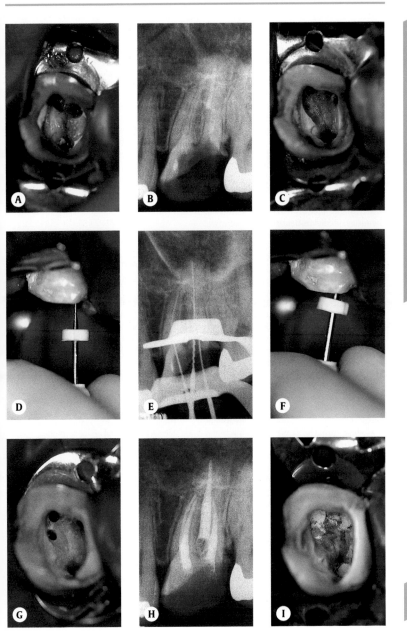

Methylene blue ($C_{16}H_{18}ClN_3S$) exists as a dark green powder or in the form of dark green, bronze-like glistening crystal. It exists in various hydrate forms and may contain up to 22% water; most common is the trihydrate.

One part methylene blue dissolves in ca. 25–40 parts water, 65 parts ethanol, or 450 parts chloroform. The substance is not soluble in diethyl ether. A 1% solution in water is acidic (pH 3–4.5). The crystals melt at 100–110°C.

Methylene blue is a nitrogen acceptor; in reversible reactions, the dye becomes a colorless leukomethylene blue, in which the previous quinoid, mesomeric-stabilized system is broken.

Methylene blue is used extensively in chemistry, medicine, dentistry, and industrial dye techniques. It is even used as a vital dye (according to Ehrlich), e.g., it stains certain histologic structures intensively and others not at all. Methylene blue stains bacteria and protozoa (blood smears according to Löffler), and is a constituent of the Giemsa and May–Grünwald histologic stains.

It also acts as an antidote (antitoxin) for carbon monooxide, prussic acid, nitrites, and aniline poisoning, and is also effective with other methemoglobin formers, because methylene blue accelerates the reduction of methemoglobin.

Methylene blue is also an antiseptic (wound rinsing, mucosal applications), antirheumatic as well as in veterinary medicine a constituent of preparations for the treatment of eczema, furuncle, as well as stomach and intestinal tract catarrh.

As a thiazine dye, it is used to color fibers (cotton, silk, polyacrylonitrile), wherein the methylene blue-zinc chloride double salt is employed.

In the form of special ingestible capsules, methylene blue is used for the diagnosis of functional stomach disorders.

Numerous legal statutes regulate the use of methylene blue in chemicals for foodstuffs, animal feed, and cosmetic additives, as well as its use in medical preparations.

In dentistry, methylene blue (canal blue) is indicated for caries diagnosis, but primarily for the identification of root canal orifices via staining of pulp tissue remnants, for the diagnosis of fracture lines as well as in retrograde surgery to stain the resection surfaces. This permits visualization of the canal and tissue debris that can then be completely removed, thus avoiding endodontic therapy failure.

For the detection of root canals, methylene blue is applied with a single-use pipette in the cavity and any excess is rinsed away. Subsequently, canal orifices can be easily distinguished by the presence of residual tissues vis-à-vis the lighter colored dentin. However, this technique may not be successful if the pulp chamber is obliterated.

Case Presentation

A Maxillary second premolar: In 48% of cases, only a single root canal; in 27%, two canals that join at the apex; and in 24%, two separate root canals with separate apical foramina. The radiograph reveals only one root canal, but the first premolar clearly exhibits two root segments. In such cases, one finds two canals in 62% of cases, and in 18% two canals with one foramen, and in 5% even three canals.

B The trepanation opening takes an oval outline. If one suspects two canal orifices, the trepanation is expanded buccally and palatally. A broad canal orifice is visible.

C For increased discernment, methylene blue (canal blue) is injected into the pulp cavity with a pipette, and the excess solution is evacuated.

D The cavity is carefully rinsed.

E Visual access to the trepanation opening reveals two separate canal orifices.

F Following expansion of the coronal opening with an Intro-File and Gates-Glidden drills, instrumentation is completed using the "crown-down" technique.

G Radiograph of the maxillary premolar revealing two separate root canal fillings with canals that converge at the apex.

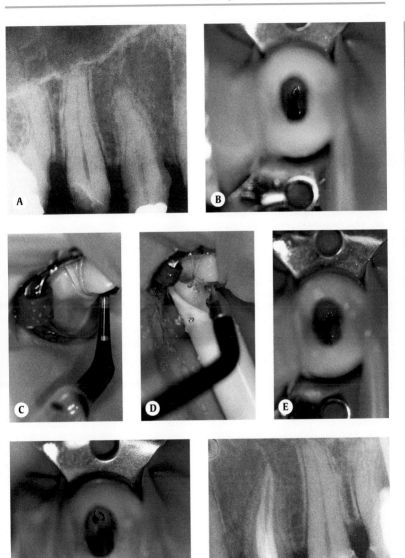

Chelators have the capacity to limit the formation of **smear layer** on the canal wall surfaces during root canal instrumentation. The effectiveness is related more to the duration of application than upon the choice of any particular preparation, and decreases significantly from coronal toward apical. Only five minutes after application there exists a 30-μm thick **demineralization zone**, which achieves 40 μm after 30 minutes and up to 50 μm after 48 hours. The interface between this layer and the subjacent dentin is a clear line of demarcation. An EDTA solution does not penetrate diffusely into dentin, rather its effect is self-limiting. Following complex formation with calcium, certain equilibrium is established so that no further dissociation occurs. Even after five days, maximum penetration is only 0.28 mm. In combination with instrumentation, chelators can significantly enhance dentin removal and therefore simplify the root canal instrumentation process.

The demineralization effect is limited however. It appears to be dependent upon the width of the root canal because, especially in narrow canals, insufficient demineralizing substance can be applied.

During instrumentation, there exists upon the internal canal wall surfaces a 5-μm thick smear layer. The depth of the densely packed **dentinal tubuli** extends up to an additional 40 μm. Constituents of the smear layer include ground dentin and pulpal tissue residues, as well as bacteria in some cases. EDTA dissolves the inorganic component of the smear layer. In combination with NaOCl, the cleansing effect is significantly increased. The use of ultrasonics does not improve cleaning efficiency further.

Following dissolution of the smear layer with EDTA, dentin permeability increases because of enlargement of the orifices of the dentinal tubuli. This results in an enhancement of the efficacy of medicament dressings in the root canal. Especially before placing calcium hydroxide dressings, the canal should be rinsed for three minutes with EDTA.

Following EDTA treatment, calcium phosphate crystals form in the depth of dentinal tubuli; these effectively close the tubuli and reduce permeability.

EDTA also possesses a slight antibacterial potential. The antibacterial effect is enhanced by a combination of EDTA and 5% NaOCl. The antibacterial effect of gel-type chelators, such as RC Prep, Glyde, or File-Care, is primarily due to the addition of 10% urea or carbamide peroxide, and depends upon the length of time the preparation is actually in contact with canal wall dentin.

Instrumentation of the root canal should always be performed using a gel-type chelator. Because of the improved cleaning efficiency and the additional antibacterial effects, a 10% peroxide additive is recommended. The paste-type chelators also serve simultaneously as a **lubricant** for the files and reduce the risk of instrument fracture. A final rinsing with 17% EDTA removes the smear layer and dramatically increases the **antibacterial effect** of interim dressings. Rinsing with a chelator is also highly recommended before removal of broken instruments or silver points from the root canal.

Case Presentation

A The initial radiograph clearly shows that the measurement instrument has penetrated only into the coronal third of the root canal, because it is very narrow.

B/C Using circumferential filing, the canal is carefully widened. There is little danger of blockage during this initial instrumentation phase.

D/E Recommended chelators include Calcinase Slight (without peroxide additive), RC Prep, Glyde, or File Care, the latter containing a 10% carbamide peroxide additive; this provides a certain bleaching effect in addition to the antibacterial effect.

F/G Through the rotating instrumentation of the root canal using the balanced-force technique, dentin chips are loosened and must be removed from the canal. Rinsing with sodium hypochlorite solution after every instrument change removes dentin chips and activates the peroxide in the chelator.

H Post-endodontic radiograph.

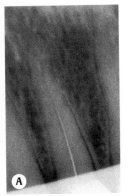

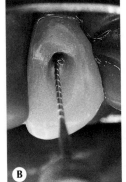

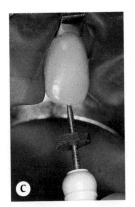

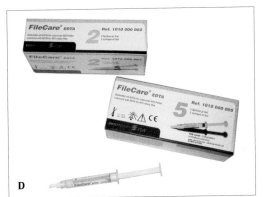

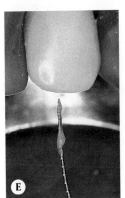

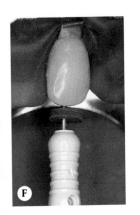

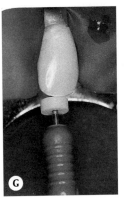

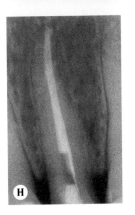

It is not possible to better discern fine details by simply moving closer to the object. If the object is too close to the eyes, it can no longer be sharply focused because of the limited **accommodation capacity**. Adults can discern objects sharply up to a distance of about 10 cm. The eyes quickly tire at this distance however. Only when the object is at 25 cm can it be clearly and sharply viewed without stress over a long period. This distance (25 cm) is called the **conventional sight distance**. At this distance, the observer can differentiate details that are approximately 0.15 mm removed from each other. This corresponds to a visual angle of two minutes. However, at such a tiny visual angle, no small details can be perceived.

In a **microscope**, the object under examination is first received from the objective and then projected further. The tube lens projects an intermediate picture that is received by the ocular and magnified for the observer's eyes. The resulting visual angle is therefore much larger.

Stereoscopic vision via the **surgical microscope** is based on the fact that, as a result of the intraocular distance, the direction of gaze upon the object is different for each eye, and therefore the two retinal images are not identical. Only in the brain of the observer are the images fused into a coherent picture with appropriate spatial relationships. With three-dimensional objects, the creation of stereoscopic effect is only possible within the **depth of focus**, and for this reason the OP microscope can only be used for slight magnification.

The introduction of the OP microscope into the field of endodontics provided improved visualization of the treatment field, i.e., the small trepanation openings or the retrograde surgical site, and made possible the most careful handling of the involved tissues in the surgical field of operation.

Using an OP microscope, the clinician will be able to discern root canal orifices that are not always possible to visualize using loupes, and seldom with the naked eye. Detecting and revealing root canals using the OP microscope demands a completely new ergonomics of instrument utilization. In both the maxilla and the mandible, the operator works with indirect vision in the 12 o'clock position, using a front-surface rhodium mirror. Working time is significantly increased.

For improved vision, the field of operation must be frequently dried; indicated for this procedure is the specially developed suction-rinse tip (Stropko, EIE, USA); the air syringe must **never** be employed.

Only after **trepanation** of the pulp chamber, is the OP microscope brought into position to locate the canal orifices. The greatest advantage is realized especially for finding all canal orifices in maxillary first molars. For example, an optical aid identified a fourth canal adjacent to the mesiobuccal canal (the so-called mesiopalatal canal) in 51% of patients. Using the microscope, a further 32% of examined teeth exhibited a fourth canal. Following extraction of the 39 teeth in this study and their histologic examination, it was demonstrated that in 90% of all maxillary first molars, a fourth root canal was in evidence.

Case Presentation

A After seating an expansive mandibular anterior bridge, the canine exhibited acute symptoms. The radiograph (slight excentric projection) reveals one root canal.

B/C Using the surgical microscope at 20–25× magnification, a second canal orifice was detected lingual to the already instrumented primary canal.

D Endodontic procedure with the OPMI 111.

E Probing the second root canal with a #15 file and a chelator gel (File Care).

F Between instrument changes, the floor of the cavity is checked under 16–25× magnification. Because of better overview, instrumentation is always performed using lower magnification.

G Both root canals were connected via an isthmus, which still contained tissue debris.

H Following completion of the root canal filling, the radiograph depicts both root canals. Following treatment, the patient was pain-free.

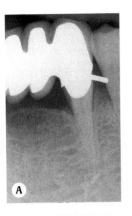

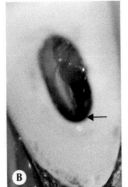

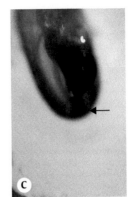

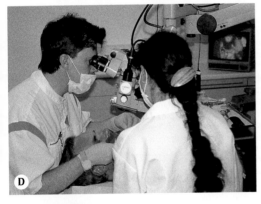

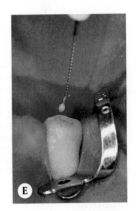

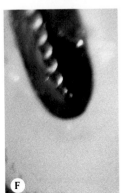

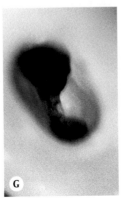

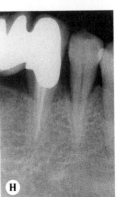

The goal of root canal instrumentation includes thorough cleansing of the canal to remove pulptissue debris, bacteria, and necrotic tissue residues, and to give the canal a shape and form that permits filling of the entire canal with a biologically inert material.

Instrumentation should be performed down to the narrowest point of the root canal, the **apical constriction**. This provides the most favorable conditions for endodontic success. In most cases, this constriction (the **physiologic foramen**) corresponds to the dentin-cementum junction; at this point, the dentin of the root canal contacts the cellular cementum of the root. The **apical foramen** is the circumferential region at the end of the root canal at which the pulpal soft tissues intertwine with the apical periodontal tissues. The dentin-cementum junction is the ideal endpoint for root canal instrumentation. Kuttler developed these criteria based on his extensive histologic study of over 400 teeth, and described precisely the location of the apical constriction and its relationship to the apical foramen. The distance between the center of the apical foramen and the apical constriction averages 0.52mm for the 25-year-old age group, and 0.66mm for the 55-year-old group.

The studies by Kuttler provided the philosophy of the **endpoint of instrumentation**. Accordingly, root canal instrumentation should end 0.5mm coronal to the radiographic apex of the root. This arbitrarily selected endpoint should prohibit any widening/opening of the apical foramen, and therefore prevent forcing bacteria into the periapical space. However, masses of bacteria from this critical apical zone are not removed by such canal length determination; thus, a periapical lesion may develop postoperatively. The critical zone is the apical 3mm of the canal. In order to eliminate bacteria and their by-products completely, it is reasonable and prudent to perform instrumentation up to the apical constriction.

Root canal instrumentation should end slightly coronal to or directly at the apex. The **anatomic apex** is the point on the tooth that is morphologically furthest removed from the incisal edge or occlusal surface; the **radiographic apex**, on the other hand, is the point furthest removed as visualized on the radiograph. The precise position can vary depending upon the anatomy of the root apex.

The **precise determination of the working length** is one of the most important procedures in endodontic treatment, and plays a major role in determining success or failure. Working length can be determined using radiographs and using electronic devices. In addition, the presence of secretions or blood on the paper point while drying the canal can provide an important clue concerning the working length. Blood on the lateral aspect of a paper point indicates a lateral perforation.

Because the precise position of apical constriction of the tooth to be treated cannot be directly ascertained from the radiograph, the tooth length is determined by measurement of the **distance from a defined coronal reference point to the radiographic apex**. This is best performed following injection of radiopaque material into the root canal. This **radiographic measurement procedure** with a #15 file within the root canal provides conclusions about root anatomy, number of root canals, as well as the course and direction of any root dilacerations.

Case Presentation

A Histologically, the apical constriction is located above the apical foramen at the level of the dentin-cementum junction. The apical foramen opens laterally, coronal to the anatomic apex. The dentin-cementum junction is not at the same level on both sides of the constriction.

B Diagnostic radiograph at initiation of root canal instrumentation. This film is viewed to ascertain an orientation of canal length.

C/D Schematic depiction of the anatomic details at the apical region, with apical constriction (2), apical foramen (3) and the radiographic apex (1). Usually the apical constriction coincides with the dentin-cementum junction (5, 6), where the dentin of the root canal and cellular cementum of the root interface.

E Within the mesiobuccal canal, the #10 file stops ca. 3mm from the apex.

F To prevent radiographic overlapping, measurement of the mesiolingual canal is performed separately.

G Final radiograph following endodontic treatment.

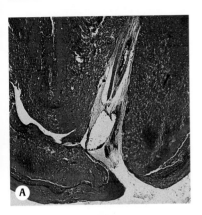

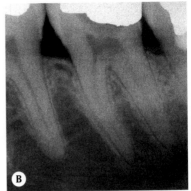

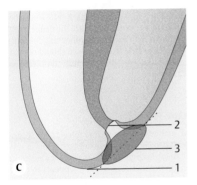

2
3
1

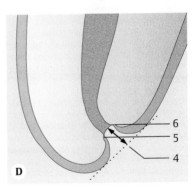

6
5
4

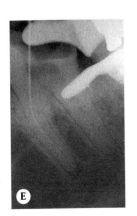

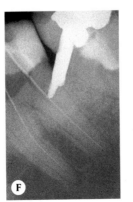

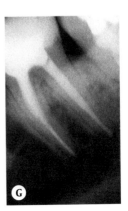

The **radiographic apex** is the only point that can be measured on a **radiograph**. In some cases, the difference between the apex and the apical constriction cannot be accurately determined. As demonstrated by Van de Voorde and Bjorndahl, the **apical constriction** is on average 1.1 mm distant from the anatomical apex and the **apical foramen** is 0.3 mm removed. Thus, the endodontic working length is only correctly determined in about 75% of cases. Forty-five percent of endodontic instruments that appear to be radiographically short of the apex actually penetrate **beyond** the apical foramen. The radiographic measurement technique does not therefore represent an arbitrary determination of the position of the physiologic foramen, but rather an approximation.

As a result of technical projection distortion, direct correction of the working length from a radiograph is scarcely possible. If the projected rays fall perpendicularly upon the root tip, the tooth will be represented somewhat enlarged. Even the right-angle radiographic technique causes a 5–7% enlargement of the true tooth length.

It is also important to remember that radiographs are not "read," but rather "interpreted." In addition to the qualities (sharpness, contrast) of the radiograph and the conditions existing during **film evaluation** (lighting, magnifying loupes), there are also subjective factors (concentration, experience, knowledge) that play important roles in radiographic evaluation. The inter-investigator agreement during evaluation of radiographs varies between 30–90%. The intra-investigator reproducibility also varies, and is often below 80%. Reproducibility by evaluation of radiographic measurements is about 70%.

During root canal instrumentation, **iatrogenic blocking** of the canal may occur inadvertently. The causes include accumulation of dentin chips that are not removed, compression of pulpal tissue debris, or the formation of an apical ledge with the accumulation of hard and soft tissues. Immediately after opening the canal orifice, a #15 Hedström file should be inserted with light rotatory movements to remove the pulpal tissues and prevent compression. Clinical experience has demonstrated that emulsification using chelator rinses during this phase of treatment dissolves pulpal tissue debris as well as the integrity of collagen fibers.

If there is any danger of **losing the appropriate working length**, it is necessary to use electronic length measurements early on, as well as additional radiographic measurement, in order to prevent additional blockage of the canal. The "traditional" concept of setting the working length just short of the apex, and then determining the working length before additional instrumentation, will lead in most cases to apical blockage. More contemporary concepts have lead to the conclusion that a patency file should be inserted to the apical endpoint to test the true traversibility of the canal, and that further instrumentation should begin with coronal expansion of the canal. Even with the use of nickel-titanium files, after each file change a #15 Hedström file should be used to prepare the deepest segments of the canal. Only following definitive working length determination should the patency file be used to determine complete root canal patency.

Case Presentation

A In the diagnostic radiograph of tooth 36, prepared using the parallel technique, a relatively large periapical radiolucency is obvious on the mesial root. There appears to be no impediment to root canal instrumentation.

B In the mesial root canals, various files were inserted for better differentiation: the K file in the mesiolingual canal has reached the working length, while the Hedström file in the mesiobuccal canal is still 2 mm too short.

C The working length was extended. Using a Hedström file of smaller size, the working depth was apparently achieved.

D/E Incorrect establishment of the working length using rubber stops leads to palpable blockage of the mesiobuccal root canal.

F The intraoperative radiograph reveals the blockage of the mesial root canals, which cannot be overcome.

G Nevertheless, three months later, the periapical radiolucency appeared smaller.

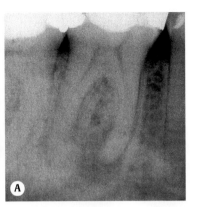

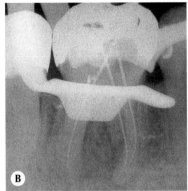

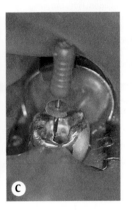

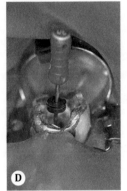

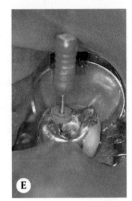

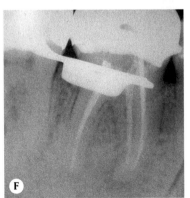

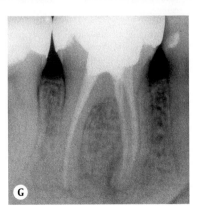

Several of the electronic devices on the market at this time integrate the measurement principle that was published in 1961 by Sunada. Using this method, the apex is considered to be achieved when the resistance between the measurement electrode and the control electrode reach a predetermined value. In teeth that have not undergone extirpation of the canal contents, there is always a resistance of 6.5 kΩ as soon as the instrument tip reaches the apex.

This principle of working length measurement defines either an absolute resistance or a resistance range. However, the tissue impedance between the apex and mucosa cannot be directly measured. If the root canal is dry all the way to the apical foramen during the measurement (which is clinically seldom possible), the measurement circuit is closed upon contact with periapical tissues. The error range increases with canal diameter; the length measurement is too long. If the root canal is moist and contains pulpal tissue debris, the predetermined resistance value will be reached short of the apex.

Considerable differences have been reported when comparing the electronically determined **canal length** with radiographically determined values. Radiographically, in 88.5% of cases the canal length will be precisely measured, while with electronic measurement the figure is only 73.1%. In dry root canals, the number of correct measurement values ranged from 67–90%; in ethanol-filled canals precise measurements were obtained in 50–73% of cases, depending on the type of instrument employed, and with NaOCl-filled canals, 37–73%.

The newest generation of electronic devices incorporate relative **impedance measurement**. In this method, two absolute impedances measured at two different frequencies are calculated by computer to achieve the absolute relationship. The electrode impedance is employed on the measurement instrument tip as a reference magnitude to determine the working length.

Electrode impedance within the root canal is high (from low current flow over the instrument tip due to the profile of the root canal) and dependent upon the profile surface of the root canal. The maximum is achieved at the apical constriction (the smallest root canal profile = largest ohm and capacitive resistance).

With further penetration of the instrument, it suddenly becomes smaller (elevated current flow in all directions). Because the dentin of the root canal wall is not an insulator, only one point in the region between the apical constriction and the apical foramen can be determined.

Any fluid within the root canal now becomes an advantage, and significantly improves the measurement results. Therefore, the root canal must be rinsed with NaOCl solution before the measurement, but the trepanation opening should be dried using a cotton pellet.

With the most contemporary devices (Root ZX, Raypex 4), the measured electrode impedance is determined over impedance quotients and is only insignificantly influenced by any electrolytes in the root canal.

In a recent publication, Hör compared electronic and radiographic working-length measurements. The contact interval for the region between the apical constriction and the apical foramen lay at 82%. On the other hand, in only 51% of cases could the apical constriction be localized precisely. Under clinical conditions, endometric devices of most recent generations appear to be capable of precisely determining the point between apical constriction and apical foramen with increased probability.

Case Presentation

A/B Using a clamp, a root canal instrument is attached to the endometric device. Via the file, the electric current is guided into the root canal; the control electrode is applied to the lip or hand.

C–E Maxillary lateral incisor with a necrotic pulp, but without clear signs of any periapical radiolucency. Root canal length can be appropriately measured in 88.5% of cases using radiography, and in 73.1–82% electronically, depending upon the commercial device.

F Using the battery-powered handpiece TriAutoZX, the working length can be determined electrometrically during canal instrumentation. When the apical constriction is encountered, the motor changes its direction of rotation and therefore determines the working length.

G Clinical application of the TriAutoZX.

H Final radiographic appearance.

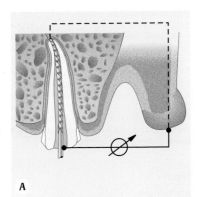

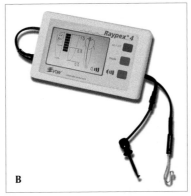

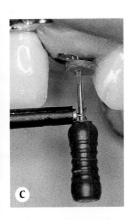

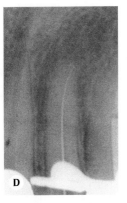

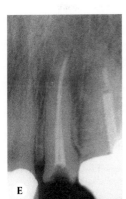

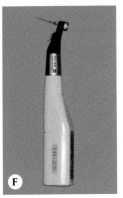

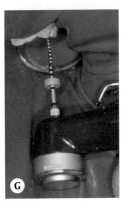

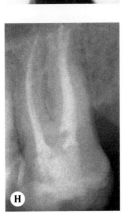

All instruments take their origins from three basic forms: **K files**, **reamers**, and **Hedström files**. The instruments were originally made from carbon steel, but since the 1960s, Cr-Ni stainless steel has been employed. Instrument lengths, strengths, dimensions, tolerances, and minimum requirements for mechanical resistance are defined by ISO standards. The diameter of the instrument tip corresponds to its size expressed in hundredths of a millimeter. The length of the progressively larger working section is 16 mm, regardless of the total instrument length. The working segment of all instruments is conical, and the diameter increases by 0.02 mm per linear mm, i.e., at the coronal-most part of the working area, the instruments are 0.32 mm thicker. For a size #15, this means that the instrument tip has a diameter of 0.15 mm and 1 mm up the shaft the diameter is 0.17 mm (0.15 + 0.02). Newer instruments made from **nickel-titanium** exhibit, in addition to the 0.02 conicity, also greater increasing diameter instruments: e.g., 04, 06, 10, and 12. Fabrication without measurement tolerances is technically impossible. The **ISO standard** permits deviations of 0.02 mm. Unfortunately, however, tolerance measurements exhibit 7–40% deviations outside the tolerance limits, depending upon manufacturer.

For easy identification and use, the instrument handles are color coded. The color codes begin with white (#15), and then yellow (#20), red (#25), blue (#39), green (#35), and black (#40). This color sequence is repeated three times up to instrument size 140. The symbol for reamers is a triangle, a square for K files, and a circle for Hedström files.

In sizes 06–25, K files are fabricated from square steel stock to increase resistance to breakage, and above size 30, triangular steel stock is used to increase flexibility. In contrast, reamers exhibit a square profile, and above size 45 triangular.

K files are manufactured by first grinding the working section from square or triangular stock, and subsequently the butt end is drilled. The individual instrument profile results from the number of windings and the cross-section of the steel. K files can also be milled out of round steel stock (e.g., Flex-R). Torsion measurements have demonstrated that breakage occurs at much higher levels in drilled instruments.

"Flexible" steel files exhibit a triangular cross-section but may also be rhomboid (K-flex). **Hedström files** are manufactured from round steel stock with progressive pitch increase, e.g., the cutting surfaces are deeper toward the instrument shaft. These are the most flexible of all steel files. The helicoid cross-section (e.g., Uniflex, S file, or Triocut files) is manufactured similarly with one cut for each two or three circular cutting edges.

Figures

A/B The cutting edge angle between the instrument axis and the cutting edge provides information about the clinical effectiveness and mechanism of action. With an angle <45˚, the rotating-scraping technique is recommended. This is especially true for reamers, which are used with a pulling and rotating movement out of the canal. A square profile is more stable. With its chip space (36%), considerably less material is transported out of the canal. The triangular cross-section is more flexible and has a larger chip space (60%).

C The cross-section of an H file with milled spirals permits a chip space of 35%, and the cutting edge angle is 60–65˚.

D After insertion of K files into the canal, circular as well as up and down movements are used to remove dentin.

E Following insertion of the Hedström file, dentin is removed using light quarter turns and apical-coronal movements circumferentially.

F Reamers are used with right or left counter-clockwise rotation as well as up and down movements.

G Special form of a Gates drill, as well as the new nickel-titanium files exhibiting more severe conicity.

H The simple helicoid cross-section of the Hedström file is exhibited as a double helix in the S file.

I NiTi files exhibit a U-shaped or a modified triangular cross-section.

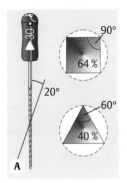

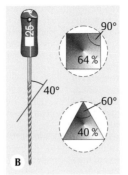

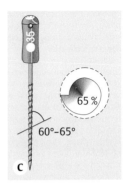

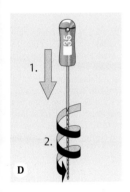

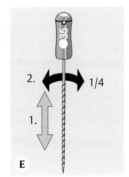

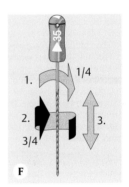

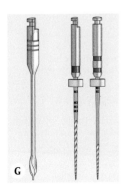

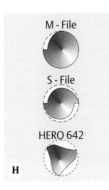

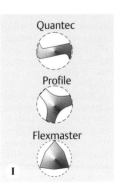

The most important characteristics of the flexibility and fracture resistance of endodontic instruments include **bending moment**, **torsion**, and **deflection**.

During instrumentation of dilacerated root canals, the **bending properties** are of critical significance. Prebending an instrument to correspond with the course of the canal brings with it an initial elastic deformation and a plastic deformation. Following such deformation, the instrument does not return to its original shape. This corresponds to the **bending moment**. Every plastic deformation leads to increased stiffness and brittleness of metals. However, any increase in brittleness signifies a reduction of plastic deformability up to and including instrument fracture. Any instrument that has been plastically deformed to conform to the root canal must not be bent back to its original shape and must never be used again because the danger of breakage will be significantly increased.

The most important **safety criterion** for cutting instruments is torsion, which measures the forces during **torsion** of the instrument. Before an instrument breaks, its profile changes by rotation in the clockwise direction. An instrument that is deformed in this way should never be reused. The behavior is dependent upon the instrument's cross-sectional profile.

With its square cross-section, reamer #35 achieves a torsion value of 159 Ncm, while reamer #45 with its triangular cross-section achieves only 139 Ncm, and is therefore more subject to fracture. K files of size 25 (square) achieve a value of 81 Ncm, the Flexicut with a triangular cross-section only 38 Ncm. Steel instruments with a higher flexibility also exhibit a higher danger of breakage.

The highest demand on an endodontic instrument is its cutting efficiency, which determines dentin removal from the internal root canal surface. As one would expect, Hedström files exhibit the best dentin removal, while square reamers are the least effective. H files (VDW) have about a 14× better cutting efficiency than K files. H files, with three circumferential cutting edges, are surprisingly less efficient than classical Hedström files. With repeated use, however, the degree of sharpness decreases dramatically. After five uses, Hedström files lose up to 80% of their cutting efficiency, K files only about 55%. Steel endodontic instruments should be considered single-use instruments, and should in no case be used more than three times.

Sterilization in the autoclave or with hot air has no effect on the cutting efficiency of stainless steel instruments.

Since 1988, endodontic instruments have been fabricated from nickel–titanium. This alloy has a low modulus of elasticity (33%, in contrast to stainless steel), and is referred to as "pseudoelastic," i.e., NiTi instruments offer only little resistance to mechanical pressure and are easily bent without incurring irreversible deformation. Because of this characteristic, these instruments can also be used mechanically in severely dilacerated root canals without the risk of immediate instrument breakage.

The cutting efficiency is dependent upon the instrument's cross-sectional profile. Instruments that exhibit a modified triangular cross-section penetrate significantly deeper into simulated root canals compared with instruments with a broad cutting surface and a U-shaped cross-section. In addition, the best cutting instruments also have the most favorable closure characteristics. Overall, however, NiTi files have lower cutting values than stainless steel files.

Figures

A Reamers (VDW, Kerr, Maillefer).

B K files

C Hedström files

D Flexicut (A), Flexofile (B), Fexoreamer (C), K-Flex (D) with rhomboid cross-section.

E Tempered tip of a Flex-R file.

F Hedström file (helicoid cutting).

G Power-driver NiTi files (Profile) with different ISO standardization and 4% conicity.

H NiTi-GT in 06, 08, 10, and 12 conicities.

I NiTi Flexogate with a 2-mm long working section, similar to Gates-Glidden.

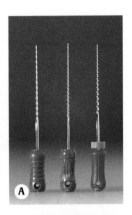

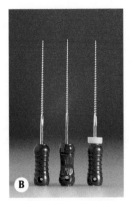

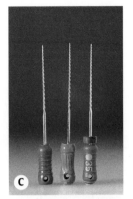

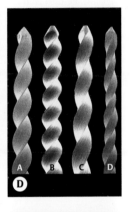

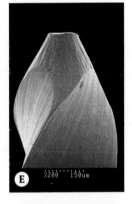

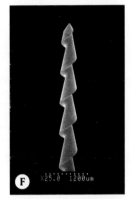

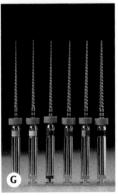

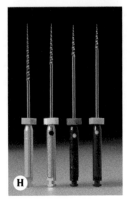

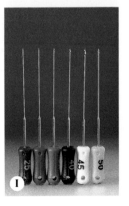

For more than a century, articles have been published regarding power-driven root canal instrumentation. The Giromatic from Micro-Mega was the accepted product after an extensive phase of development. Nevertheless, it had several disadvantages: The hoped for time saving was only slight, the fine tactility of hand instruments was often lost, dilacerated root canals were often "straightened" and the walls were inadequately smoothed. Errors of instrumentation in dilacerated canals led to funnel formation or even perforation of the canal wall.

The mechanical mechanisms used in today's power-driven endodontics include a **90˚ rotation** (Giromatic, Endocursor, IntraEndoLift), combinations with a **hub movement** (EndoLift), lateral movement (Excalibur), as well as **hub plus rotation** (IntraEndo 3 LDSY and Canal Leader).

In 1984, Levy developed the Canal Finder; it combined the RPM-dependent hub movement with a slipping clutch that released if the friction of the file within the canal became too great. Using special H files with rounded tips, a helicoid motion resulted. The new Canal Leader exhibits a 30˚ rotation with 0.4-mm hub movement, both of which are dependent upon resistance within the canal. However, this device also has weaknesses, as with other power-driver systems.

Efforts were also made to incorporate **sonic or ultrasonic vibrations** for root canal instrumentation. In 1976, Martin and Cunningham described the use of "magnetostriction" for the piezoelectric effect to create vibrations of 20 000–40 000 Hz. Shortly thereafter, sonic vibration systems were introduced that could convert the compressed air from the dental unit to frequencies up to 6000 Hz.

All of these systems occasioned transversal oscillation of the canal instrument; however, these were dampened as soon as the instrument was pressed onto the canal wall or became bound within the canal. Therefore, small instruments are more effective than large ones, and sonic waves are advantageous because they exhibit larger amplitude than ultrasound under longitudinal loading of the instrument tip. In addition, problems such as ledge formation and instrument fracture are less. However, with both systems, the shaping of a dilacerated root canal is not optimum. With ultrasound, microacoustic streaming with small primary vortices and larger secondary vortices create forces that can destroy bacteria and tissue debris when in the presence of a rinsing solution. The cleansing and disinfecting effect of the combination of ultrasound and sodium hypochlorite is superior to all other methods. Unfortunately, the actual instrumentation is attended by problems of surface roughness, shape changes, and canal blockage. Ultrasonic devices have recently found new areas of use including microinstruments in retrosurgery and diamond-coated tips for widening the canal orifice.

Still today, the **Gates-Glidden** drills remain the universal instruments for power-driven endodontic therapy; these are used both for coronal widening of the root canal and also for revision of restorative materials.

Nickel-titanium alloys have long been used in orthodontics. Their positive characteristics such as low modulus of elasticity, high deflective capability, shape, "memory," and superelasticity made this alloy the material of choice. With the development of nickel-titanium endodontic instruments since 1988, a new generation of files has been created whose flexibility significantly simplifies the difficult instrumentation of dilacerated canals. In comparison to steel files, changes in the course of a root canal are less pronounced using NiTi files. Even the shape of the files leads more often to a round canal cross-section.

Figures

A Gates-Glidden drills sizes 50, 70, 90, 110, 130, and 150.

B Gates drill and special shapes (Largo, Peeso).

C EndoLift, Giromatic, Canal Leader.

D Power-driven instruments: Lentulos (left), K files (middle), and Hedström files (right).

E Reamer, H files, and K files (SEM photo).

F Sonic-Air attachment with Kerr sonic file.

G Instruments for sonic and ultrasonic devices.

H Shaper and Rispisonic with concentric spiral hooks; ultrasonic files with K design.

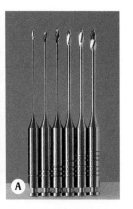

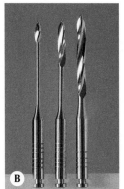

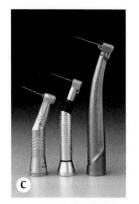

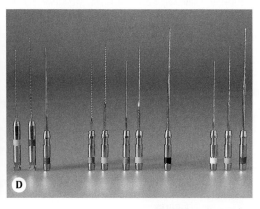

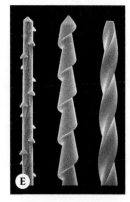

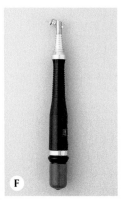

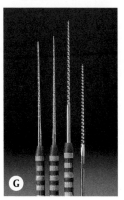

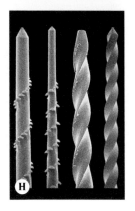

These two terms, cleaning and shaping, encompass and characterize clearly the most **basic requirements** for canal instrumentation, which were established by the "old master" of endodontics, Professor Schilder, more than 30 years ago: cleansing and giving the canal a proper form to receive the filling.

Cleaning signifies the removal of all materials from the root canal, including infiltrated tissues, antigenic material, all organic components, bacteria and their products, but also caries, tissue debris as well as denticles and other hard tissue accumulations, contaminated canal filling material and other inflammation-inducing agents. Cleaning also means the **instrumentation** and mechanical removal of canal constituents, chemical dissolution of tissue debris, and rinsing them out of the canal.

Shaping is the **creation** of a special cavity shape, and includes five requirements (see below). This "shape" for the radicular preparation of the tooth makes it possible to freely insert pluggers, spreaders, or other obturation instruments and to apply sufficient force to those instruments, ultimately to permit the seating of a well-formed gutta percha point. A perfectly shaped gutta percha point also leads in the ideal case to the complete closure of lateral canals and all canal irregularities. This makes possible a three-dimensional closure of the entire root canal system. Shaping is the mechanical part of root canal instrumentation and is achieved through the proper use of Gates-Glidden drills, slow speed burs, ultrasonic and sonic devices, hand instruments, and not least of all use of the new nickel-titanium instruments with appropriate conicity (e.g., shaping files).

The first step toward successful cleaning and shaping is a **coronal access** of sufficient expanse. In addition to the **apical shape**, the "**body**" **shape** and the "**taper**" (conicity) toward the apex are of great importance. There remains some controversy regarding the designation of the apical opening: Schilder called it "foraminal patency," by which the passage through the canal apex was guaranteed by the passage of a thin K file through the canal and slightly beyond the apical foramen during instrumentation.

The **five requirements concerning canal shape** (Schilder, 1974) are:

- establish a continually widening conical root canal shape from apex to coronal
- establish in the region of the apex a very narrow canal with the smallest diameter at the apical termination
- divide any dilacerated canal into several levels, and prepare separately each of the multiple levels
- do not ever alter the position of the apical foramen in the lateral direction
- maintain the apical foramen as small as necessary during the instrumentation process.

Instrumenting the canal to #20 or #25 (seldom to #30), is sufficient at the apical foramen, so that the apical constriction is not unnecessarily expanded. A continuously expanding canal shape beginning with preparation at the coronal aspect, as well as adequate rinsing, is important for success. The majority of infected and necrotic tissue is always localized to the coronal and middle third of the canal. This area should be instrumented first, and sufficiently expanded laterally. Repeatedly, the previous file should be reinserted, or a #15 K file or H file should be used to prevent any possible blockage of the canal.

Figures

A The shape of the canal is clearly conical and widened coronally. In the apical third, only minimal widening; via patency, canal blockage is prevented.

B With inadequate prebending of the instruments, the apical foramen is "transported" and ledges created.

C Initial perforation: creation of a ledge.

D Inappropriate widening of the apical dilaceration caused by inadequate or incorrect prebending of the instrument.

E The consequence is the creation of a step, bordering on perforation.

F Complete perforation in the apical region.

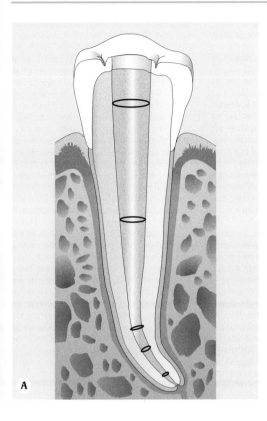

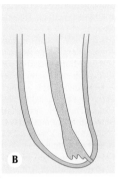

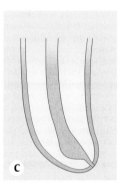

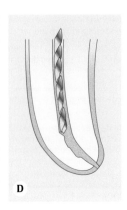

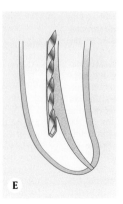

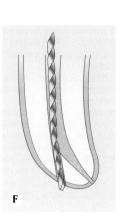

One differentiates between the apical-coronal and the coronal-apical instrumentation techniques:

- Using the **apical-coronal technique**, the apical region is first completely instrumented, and then the root canal is conically instrumented in the coronal direction. This technique creates an apical stop, and forms the root canal slightly diverging toward the pulp chamber. In this technique, there are two different methods of instrumentation: the step-back technique and the standardized technique.
- In contrast, when using **coronal-apical instrumentation**, first the coronal segment of the canal is widened and then the apical region of the canal is instrumented.

Using the **step-back technique**, the apical region is initially instrumented and subsequently the coronal aspect of the root canal is shaped. Immediately after trepanation, a radiograph is used to determine the working length. The first file that is set to the working length and inserted into the canal to the point it binds is referred to as the **initial apical file**, IAF. The root canal must be conically widened with this IAF file and four sequentially larger instruments. During this initial phase of instrumentation, no instrument size must be skipped because of the danger of blocking the canal. It is recommended to **reinsert** the previous file to insure the quality of instrumentation to the proper depth. Following each change of instrument, the canal must be copiously rinsed.

The final file that is used at the working length, and which continues to remove white dentin chips, is referred to as the **apical master file**, AMF. Its size corresponds later to the gutta percha master point.

The coronal portion of the root canal is subsequently conically shaped using the step-back technique through four additional instruments sizes. To accomplish this, the four final files are adjusted 1 mm shorter than the AMF, which provides the ascending conical canal configuration with a defined apical stop. A final traverse with the apical master file will ensure the patency of the root canal.

In one study, the cleanliness of the root canal as well as its course and form were studied following instrumentation with K files, Hedström files, and Unifiles. The results demonstrated that only the K files used in the step-back technique provided a definitive apical stop, an almost round canal cross-section, a very good apical preparation without any indentations, as well as a conical canal shape from apical toward coronal. With dilacerated canals, however, in 46% of cases the apical course of the canal was altered.

The instrumentation of straight root canals is performed clockwise, i.e., with right rotation (reaming). Such instrumentation is not without risk. During the **rotatory movements**, the file's cutting edges cut deeply into dentin and this can lead to wedging of the instrument and binding in the canal. During instrumentation and when removing it from the root canal, the instrument shaft can fracture. If the root canal is slightly dilacerated, ledges may be cut internally, resulting in loss of the true working length. When using K files with a rotatory working stroke, a round root canal cross-sectional profile will be achieved 1 mm coronal to the foramen in 80% of cases. If the radius of curvature is increased, the number of truly round preparation shapes will be simultaneously reduced: With a curvature radius > 25°, only 33% will be round. At the apical level, a round canal profile will only be achieved using a size 40 instrument.

Case Presentation

A Determining the working length.

B After determining the IAF (#20), the canal is further enlarged by four sizes to the AMF (#40).

C The first files (#45 and #50) following the AMF are adjusted 1 mm and 2 mm shorter.

D The third file after the AMF (#55) is set 3 mm shorter. The final file (#60) is termed the final file (FF).

E The radiograph taken three months later depicts a homogeneous filling, but only slight conicity.

F After instrumenting the root canal up to the apical master file (here, size 35), the following files are adjusted 1 mm shorter. This provides an optimum ascending conicity of the root canal form. The various stages are interrupted by regular use of the apical master file for smoothing the root canal surfaces.

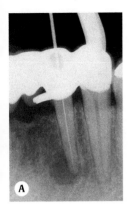

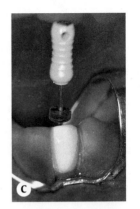

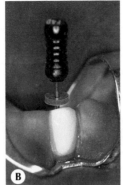

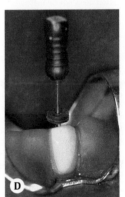

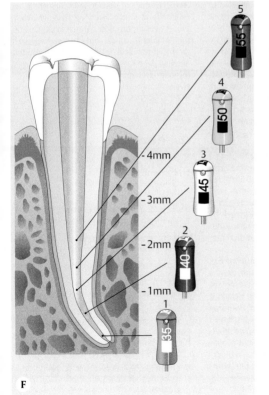

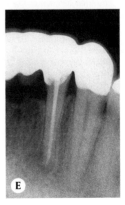

119

Using this technique, the coronal portion of the root canal is instrumented first, and then the apical region. An **advantage** of this technique vis-à-vis the apical-coronal technique is that the rinsing cannula can be inserted deeply into the coronal opening to ensure adequate rinsing of the root canal during instrumentation. During instrumentation of the apical region, necrotic pulpal tissues are better loosened by the NaOCl rinse.

To begin the procedure, it is necessary to determine the apical patency of the root canal. To accomplish this, a #15 file is used initially with one-eighth turns and light pressure in the root canal. By means of circumferential filing, the canal is carefully widened; blockage of the canal in this initial phase of instrumentation need not be feared.

Thereafter, a **Gates-Glidden drill** is used to expand the coronal aspect of the canal up to the point of any dilaceration. The Gates drill (size 1, #50) widens the canal up to the dilaceration at 500 rpm, and the tip of the instrument is coated with a lubricant. The Gates drill size 2 (#70) is adjusted 1 mm shorter; sizes 3, 4, and 5 each 1 additional mm shorter.

Frequent and copious rinsing with sodium hypochlorite solution following each instrument usage will rinse dentin chips out of the canal.

Following **coronal expansion**, the working length is determined radiographically using a size 15 K file. If the narrowness of the root canal does not permit introduction of the K file to the working depth, a Hedström file must be carefully employed to create the necessary space.

Apical instrumentation is performed by means of circumferential filing with Hedström files and then rotationally with K files (balanced force).

Thereafter, using a size 20 Hedström file, the coronal aspect is widened, and then a prebent K file of size 20 is used to instrument the entire root canal to the working length. If the file cannot be inserted to the working length, the instrument should not be forced apically with rotation. If this occurs, the previous file should be reapplied. Through proper use of a **patency file**, the danger of canal blockage or ledge creation is for the most part eliminated, and the canal dilaceration can be successfully traversed.

According to the canal's degree of dilaceration, the instruments must be appropriately prebent in order to avoid any funnel shape at the apex. The bending should be made only in the apical portion of the instrument; any bending of the instrument further coronally can lead to undesired **straightening** of the canal.

Following determination of the initial apical file, the root canal is enlarged four additional file sizes up to the apical master file, in this case size 35.

This technique prevents transfer of bacteria from the coronally infected root canal segments into apical, noninflamed areas, because the initial procedure removes necrotic and infected tissues from the coronal and middle canal segments. This accounts for the fact that the occurrence of post-endodontic pain is significantly less than after the step-back technique. In addition, after coronal expansion using Gates drills, apical root canal segments are tactily better achieved. The rinsing cannula extends deep into the root canal and the rinsing supports manual instrumentation effectively.

Case Presentation

A Using increasingly larger Gates-Glidden drills, the coronal and middle canal segments are initially enlarged to the point of the canal dilaceration.

B Thereafter, the canal is enlarged to the working length using prebent hand instruments.

C Determining the patency of the coronal preparation.

D Coronal expansion using Gates-Glidden drills of increasing diameter.

E Determining the precise working length.

F Establishing the initial apical file (#15), i.e., the first file that binds at working length.

G Using careful rotatory motions, the root canal is widened along its entire length.

H The radiograph depicts the increasing conicity of the root canal filling from apical toward coronal.

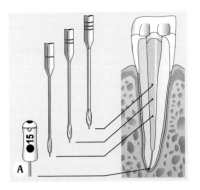

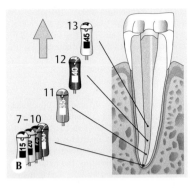

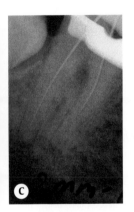

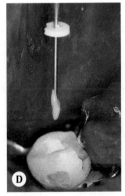

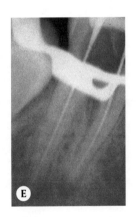

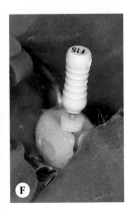

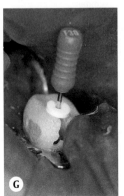

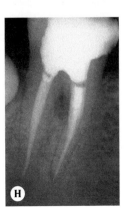

Following trepanation and extirpation of the pulpal tissues, the working length is determined radiographically. The double-flare technique involves three procedures:
1. reverse flaring
2. apical instrumentation
3. flaring of the entire root canal.

The canal orifice is an anatomically determined narrowing, the "coronal constriction." Early elimination of this constriction simplifies the subsequent instrumentation steps. **Coronal widening** is performed via **"reverse flaring."** To accomplish this, the hand instruments (files) destined for later apical instrumentation are employed in reverse order. After using a #15 K file to determine the entire length and the course of the canal, a #45 K file is used only in the first few millimeters of the coronal portion of the canal; subsequently a #40 file is applied deeper in the coronal region, and a #35 K file is used to instrument still deeper in the apical direction.

After coronal widening of the area of the canal orifice up to the middle of the canal, the #15 K file is again used to the **full working length** to widen the entire root canal; this is followed by files #17, 20, 22, 25, and 27. The clinician can either use Golden–Medium files (Maillefer) as intermediate sizes in addition to the standard sizes 15, 20, and 25, or one can "fabricate" these files in the operatory by shortening the instrument tips by appropriate millimeter length. Because the cross-sectional diameter of a K file with 2% conicity per millimeter in length increases by 0.02mm, a corresponding trimming of the instrument tip will create an intermediate size. The shortened tip is sharp but irregular and must be smoothed using a diamond-coated file. Subsequently the instrument is sterilized in the hot bead sterilizer.

After completion of the **apical widening** up to size 30, a **step-back technique** at size 35 is used, but shorter by 1 mm. Subsequently, the previous instrument file is again used to the complete working length in order to prevent canal blockage. Size 40 is shortened by 2mm, size 45 by 3mm, and size 50 by 4mm; this creates a conical "flaring" within the apical third of the canal.

In addition to the procedure described above, coronal widening can also be accomplished using Hedström files or the Gates–Glidden drills. In addition, shaping files from the ProTaper System are indicated.

During the process of **apical instrumentation** of the root canal, the small files must be employed over a sufficient time. Within the ISO system, the relative increase in instrument diameters among the small files is significantly larger than among the larger files, percentage-wise. For example, the diameter between sizes 10 and 15 increases by 50%. Between sizes 30 and 35, the increase is only 16.7%.

In **summary**, the double-flare technique involves coronal widening, beginning with large instruments, and then smaller files are used to progress ever deeper into the canal. Then smaller instruments are used for instrumentation from apical toward coronal. Thus the procedure is **double flaring**, from coronal and from apical. As such, this technique corresponds to a combination of step-down and step-back techniques.

Case Presentation

A Initial radiograph of a maxillary second molar.

B After checking canal patency, a #35 K file is used to initiate the coronal expansion by using the instrument circumferentially.

C A smaller file (size 30) extends about 2mm deeper into the root canal.

D The "double flaring" of the root canal is divided into two procedures: One begins with larger files in the coronal root canal segment, and then smaller files progress ever deeper into the canal.

E At the full working length, the canal is enlarged through four instruments sizes, and then flaring in the coronal direction is performed as with the step-back technique.

F/G After apical shaping, the coronally directed instrumentation is depicted; the K file #40 is shortened by 2mm and the #45 by 3mm.

H Note the conical shape of the root canal filling.

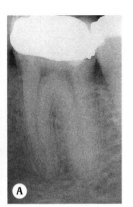

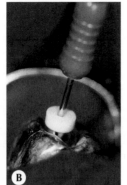

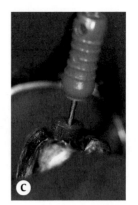

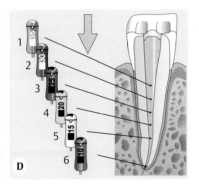

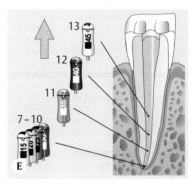

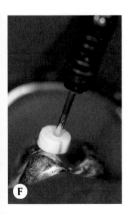

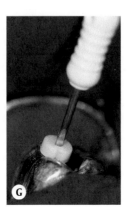

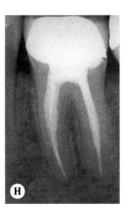

In contrast to the step-down technique, one begins with larger instruments in the coronal region of the root canal when using this instrumentation method. Following this **coronally initiated instrumentation**, smaller files penetrate ever deeper into the canal until the smallest files achieve the root apex. Nevertheless, in every case the #15 K file is used to determine the patency of the entire root canal length.

Following coronal expansion, the working length is determined radiographically using a #15 file. Deviations of more than 2 mm from the established working depth are not immediately corrected but only after instrumentation of the coronal and middle thirds of the canal, using a second radiographic measurement.

One initiates the **coronal widening** with a #35 K file; this will only penetrate a few millimeters into the coronal aspect of the canal, which is then widened carefully by circumferential filing. The canal is then rinsed and a #15 file is used to test further canal patency. The repeated use of the #15 file is extraordinarily important in order to prevent canal blockage. Then a #30 file is used to penetrate a few millimeters deeper; subsequent use of the #15 file is also necessary, to penetrate into the middle third of the root canal. The #20 file proceeds deeper; careful circumferential filing proceeds to widen this segment of the canal. Using the #15 file, one finally achieves the apical segment, a #10 file is inserted still deeper, and a #08 file finally reaches the apical constriction.

With reference to the diagnostic radiograph, the files must be carefully prebent. The Flexobend (Maillefer) is used for prebending; the plastic rollers permit bending of the instrument at virtually any point without damage to the cutting edges and without buckling. If the files are not prebent, triangular files will remove material from the external aspect of a dilacerated canal at the apical area. This leads to a pouch-shaped alteration of the canal. The working length is reduced by up to 2.4 mm.

Files that are prebent to correspond with root canal anatomy bind in dilacerated canals only at the instrument tip, while files that are not prebent may bind along the entire length. Binding only at the tip permits improved tactile determination of any resistances.

Straight and not prebent files can be inserted into the canal only with force. This means that irregularities and dilacerations will not be recognized, and thus ledges and blockages may be created. A major problem with forceful apical insertion of instruments is that any tactile feedback is completely lost, bringing with it the loss of critically important information concerning the attainment of the apical constriction.

Following this initial instrumentation, beginning coronally, one then proceeds with the identical process using the next larger file (size 40) to expand coronally. Smaller files reach deeper, and this **second crown-down sequence** is continued to the apex with a #10 file. In a third sequence, one begins coronally with a size 45 file and achieves the apex at #15. This sequence of instrumentation is continued until the apex has been achieved with four increasingly large files, always dependent upon the first file size that achieved the apex.

In the coronal aspect, Gates-Glidden drills can also be used for rapid enlargement.

Case Presentation

A Maxillary second premolar and second molar exhibiting pulpal necrosis and periapical radiolucency.

B Initial coronal expansion, depicted here using GT manual files and a 10% conicity.

C The crown-down technique is performed in several sequences, from coronal toward apical, beginning with a #35 K file. At the apical region, file #10 achieves the constriction.

D The procedure is repeated until the apical region is widened to file #25 size. Coronally, Gates-Glidden drills can also be used for instrumentation and conical shaping.

E With GT files, files of ever smaller conicity penetrate more deeply into the canal.

F Radiographic view of the final root canal fillings.

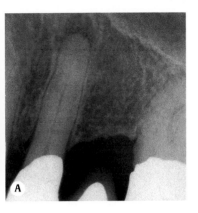

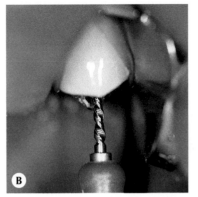

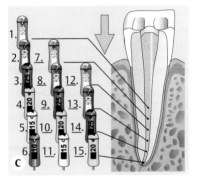

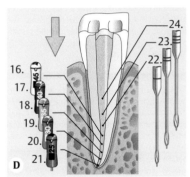

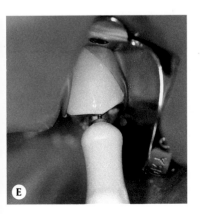

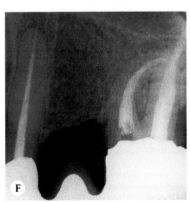

Root Canal Filling with Limited Mouth Opening

In order to avoid ledge creation or blockage in the region of the apical 4mm, the root canal instruments must be prebent. Space problems can occur when using instruments 25 and more mm long in a patient with inhibited jaw opening. Therefore, during initial instrumentation, the instrument is inserted into the mesial root canals of molars. The stopper notch will then provide orientation, first in the **mesial** canal and subsequently distally.

Apically, the instruments are more severely prebent than the actual canal dilaceration, and this is indicated by the stopper tip or notch, which initially points mesially. The instrument is inserted into the mesiobuccal canal opposite to the direction of the dilaceration. During the rest of the almost force-free progressive insertion into the root canal, the file is slowly rotated, and this can be visualized on the stopper tip; finally, the stopper tip (or notch) points **distally**.

Funnel Formation

An apical funnel will form as the result of improper instrumentation and straightening of the apical segment of a dilacerated root canal. To prevent such funnel formation, the apical end of the instrument must be bent more severely than the canal dilaceration that is visible on the radiograph. Only the use of sufficiently long, thin, and flexible files will prevent any apical widening. When using the balanced-force technique, the instrument must be removed from the canal and carefully cleaned following each rotation, and again prebent before reinsertion. Any excessively expansive apical widening **must** be avoided; as a general rule, dilacerated posterior tooth roots are only instrumented to file size 25 at the apex. Both steel and also NiTi files of this size are very flexible and therefore unlikely to alter the course of the canal.

In order to avoid excessive overinstrumentation of the outer curvature of the canal when using larger, less flexible instruments, a diamond-coated instrument is used to "dull" the file on the outer surface of the apical 3–4mm. Not every file should be dulled, rather every second file, because otherwise no dentin would be removed in the apical region.

Perforation

Aggressively excessive initial instrumentation of the mesial canals of molars can lead to a breach of the canal wall. The course of the canal must be carefully interpreted using a diagnostic radiograph. This examination will determine whether the use of Gates-Glidden drills is indicated. Hedström files up to size 25 can initially widen the root canal sufficiently. By using anticurvature filing, excessive removal of hard tissue can be avoided, i.e., distal walls are intentionally not instrumented. If the root itself is small and narrow, a paper point is inserted into the canal after the use of a size 30 file in order to ascertain any lateral bleeding. Such bleeding indicates a lateral perforation.

Overinstrumentation

This problem can be avoided by accurate radiographic working length measurement and determination of the proper apical reference point. It is important to establish a reproducible coronal reference point, which will be different for each root canal. Using electronic length determination, a length correction can be made, e.g., as a result of inadvertent or accidental straightening of dilacerated root canal segments.

Case Presentation

A/D The prebent file is inserted 180° opposite to the actual root canal dilaceration.

B/E As the file is inserted further, it is rotated 180° within the canal; this is indicated by the stopper marking.

C/F/G When the file has reached the working length, the stopper marking will point in the direction of the apical dilaceration.

H Master point radiograph (four root canals).

I Final radiograph of the root canal fillings.

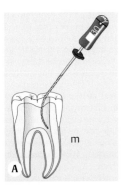

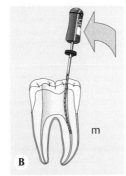

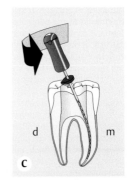

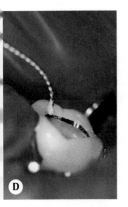

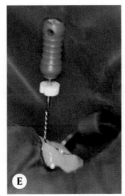

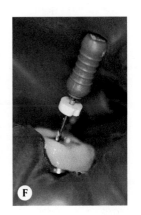

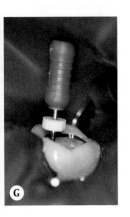

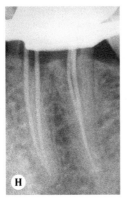

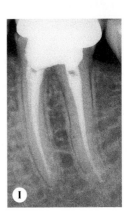

The ability of pulpal cells to form hard tissue is not limited to the odontoblastic layer. Fibrodentin accumulations also occur centrally in the form of **denticles** within the pulpal tissues in both erupted and nonerupted deciduous and permanent teeth, as well as both young and old teeth. With increasing age, more formation of intrapulpal dentin occurs, and subsequently the root canal becomes increasingly narrow. Such hard tissue formation is usually the consequence of an inflammatory process.

Fifty percent of teeth exhibiting crown fractures also exhibit such mineralizations, including lamella denticles as well as **diffuse accumulations**; inflammatory cells can be observed in 25%.

Healthy teeth in 10–20-year-olds exhibit pupal mineralizations in only 8% of patients; carious teeth from the same age group have an incidence of 36%. In the age group 45–63 years, 90% of examined teeth exhibit calcifications. Such calcifications become visible in a radiograph only when they exceed a size of 200μm.

Teeth with **degenerative calcifications** are usually symptom-free. Endodontic treatment for such teeth is extremely difficult, time-consuming, and expensive; the decision to treat must be seriously considered! In most cases, a "wait-and-see" attitude is the best approach; in rare cases, an immediate surgical procedure may be necessary. If the canal orifices cannot be detected, the cavity is rinsed and stained with methylene blue. This is often not helpful, however, because only organic tissues are stained. If the clinician suspects or knows the position of the canal orifices, they are identified by probing and opened using an **ultrasonic spreader** (with a diamond-coated tip). Because the use of ultrasonic files usually leads to a false opening, they are not indicated in cases of root canal obstructions.

EDTA can increase dentin permeability and therefore favorably influence debridement of the root canal. Because of the slow-acting effect of this hard tissue-demineralizing agent, decalcification of dentin during canal instrumentation is unlikely. For the ultimate opening of obliterated root canals, the tip of a K file is coated with a small amount of RC Prep and then inserted into the root canal using small rotatory movements. To overcome obstructions, considerable time will be required. After removal of the file from the canal, it must be carefully cleaned using sterile gauze. Then the cavity is thoroughly rinsed with NaOCl solution. This elevates dentin permeability, increases the release of oxygen, and neutralizes the EDTA.

During root canal instrumentation, unexpected and unplanned iatrogenic canal **blockage** can occur. The causes include an accumulation of dentin chips that are not successfully removed, compression of pulpal tissue debris or apical ledge formation with accumulation of hard and soft tissues. If pulpal tissues have been compressed, a lubricant must be used, even in the depth of the root canal. Only through the use of a Hedström file, size 15, with slight rotatory movements, can such tissue accumulations be successfully penetrated. The file must be repeatedly cleaned and resterilized.

If a loss of working length occurs during instrumentation, any **forceful** deeper preparation to break through the obstruction must be avoided completely.

Case Presentation

A Tooth 25 exhibits an inadequate root canal filling and a periapical radiolucency. Tooth 24 exhibits only a post build-up without canal filling; the root canal is partially obliterated.

B After chemical softening, the gutta percha is removed.

C Initial situation following trepanation of tooth 25, with apparently only one canal.

D Under the surgical microscope, two root canals are detected and subsequently instrumented.

E The post build-up on tooth 24 was loosened using ultrasonics, and the cavity was then filled with an EDTA lubricant.

F Following ultrasonic preparation, the obstruction was removed using an H file. Rinsing with citric acid followed.

G Final radiograph of the root canal fillings.

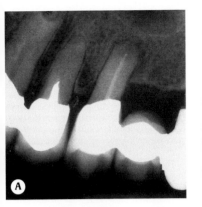

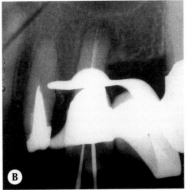

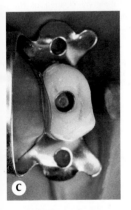

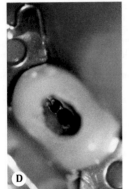

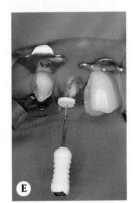

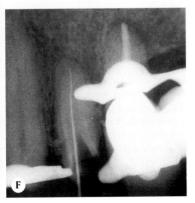

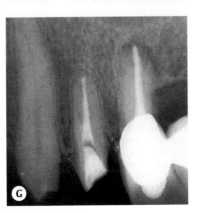

In order to relieve the dentist from some of the very laborious and time-consuming root canal instrumentation, Rollins (1899) described a needle-shaped root canal bur that was driven by a dental motor. Speed limitation to 100 rpm was intended to avoid instrument breakage. However, it was not until the introduction of the Racer file head in 1958 and the Giromatic handpiece in 1964 that the epoch of power-driven root canal instrumentation began.

The Giromatic handpiece produced reciprocating quarter turns, and was imitated by many other manufacturers. The IntraEndo 3LD utilizes alternating 80° rotations, while the Endolift 1 produces vertical strokes in addition to reciprocating one-quarter turns.

As has been shown by numerous investigations, the **Giromatic** system does not adequately instrument narrow or severely dilacerated canals, and the shaping function is also critical; usually it leads to ledge formation, to obvious deviation from the preoperative course of the canal, and even to the creation of "iatrogenic canals." Additional problems included frequent canal straightening and funnel-like formation at the apex, insufficient smoothing, and even blockage of the apical segment of the root canal. Perforations and instrument fracture also occurred. Today as always, hand instrumentation is superior to the power-driven instrumentation.

Results with the **Endolift** were not significantly different from the Giromatic. In comparison with other power-driven systems, the Endolift was characterized by removing the least amount of material. In some cases, severe straightening of dilacerated canal segments was observed, and instrument fracture was common. The surfaces of the canal walls often exhibited significant scratches and grooves.

The **Racer** was associated with the occurrence of acute painful reaction due to apical compaction and extrusion of infected dentin chips. Following instrumentation to file size 35, only two-thirds of the dilacerated root canals were adequately prepared. Straightening of the apical segment of the canal was a consistent finding.

With the **Excalibur**, the files execute multilateral movements, or so-called aleatoric oscillations. Excalibur instrumentation produced an acceptable shape in only one-third of the canals.

The primary movement of the **Canalfinder** system is a vertical stroke with amplitude that depends upon the rotational speed and the resistance offered by the canal, and usually is maximally 1 mm. With higher rpm, the amplitude decreases; beyond 2000 rpm it is only 0.3 mm. The manufacturer recommends the use of 1000–8000 rpm. A rotational movement is created by the contact of the oblique cutting edges of the instrument with the canal wall. Translational movements (up and down) and rotation together provide a helicoidal motion.

The Canalfinder also provided inadequate instrumentation of curved root canals, and regions with completely uninstrumented canal surfaces were observed. None of the canals studied were completely cleaned or thoroughly smoothed. An advantage of the Canalfinder, however, was its ability to frequently open even very narrow and severely dilacerated root canals initially, frequently even in a very short period of time.

The **Endoplaner** exhibits small, coronally directed scraping movements when the instrument is pressed against the canal wall. It simulates the Hedström file motions, and is indicated for coronal expansion using the circumferential technique.

The **reduction of tactile feedback** accompanied by **loss of working length** is common to all power-driven devices.

Case Presentation

A Diagnostic radiograph of a maxillary molar with dilacerated root canals.

B Following preparation of the access cavity, the working length is determined and adjusted.

C The mechanism of action of the Endolift 2 is a reciprocal vertical-rotatory movement. Commercially available hand instruments are employed in this device.

D During clinical use, the working length must be marked with a rubber stopper.

E The working files from the handpiece are used to check working length.

F The final radiograph reveals minimal canal straightening, loss of working depth, as well as overinstrumentation of the distobuccal canal.

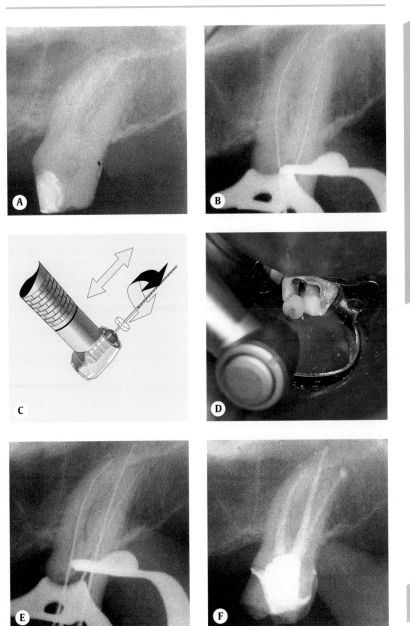

For use in endodontics, two titanium alloys have been used to date: titanium-aluminum and nickel-titanium alloys. Both of these alloys take advantage of the special characteristics of titanium; titanium combined with the primary nickel component has become the basic material for the fabrication of root canal instruments.

In addition to the titanium-aluminum alloy, presently there are four **nickel-titanium alloys** available for use as dental raw materials. These alloys are produced by numerous manufacturers, and with varying compositions:

- **Nitinol**: Ni stands for nickel, Ti for titanium, and NOL for Naval Ordinance Laboratory (Silver Spring, Maryland, USA) according to the manufacturers of the alloy. It consists of 56 m% Ni and 44 m% Ti.
- **Chinese NiTi** or **Nitalloy** with a composition of 56 m% Ni and 44 m% Ti.
- **Japanese NiTi** (Furukawa Electric, Japan).
- Nitinol amalgamated with cobalt.

Titanium-aluminum alloys for root canal instruments contain a composition of about 95 m% titanium and 5 m% aluminum.

All nickel-titanium alloys exhibit a small modulus of elasticity (33–43%, in contrast to stainless steel). Some authors characterize this property as **superelasticity** or **pseudoelasticity**, i.e., the instruments present only slight resistance to mechanical force and are easy to bend, but without irreversible deformation.

This can be explained by the **various crystal-lattice formations**: When force is applied, the austenitic structure of a nickel-titanium wire changes into a tension-induced martensite.

With increasing load, the crystal lattice achieves a plastically deformable condition. Under constant temperature conditions, a significant expansion occurs without any significant increase of tension. This is referred to as the "superelastic plateau." With reduction of tension, the metal returns to its original austenitic condition.

Another metallurgic peculiarity is the so-called **memory effect**, which is also called **shape memory**, martensitic memory, or **mechanical memory**. This quality is interdependent with the superelasticity: At a temperature of ca. 100°C, the nickel-titanium alloy exists almost exclusively in the form of the austenitic phase. With a decrease in temperature, the metallic structure reverts to a martensite, which correlates with the characteristics of the previously described superelasticity. If the nickel-titanium wire in this condition experiences a deformation, it can be eliminated at any time by heating the material to above 125°C. This property is called "**shape memory**."

In addition, titanium and to a certain extent nickel-titanium alloys possess the property of rapid passivity when exposed to corrosive media. This is an important prerequisite for the biocompatibility of any metal.

The composition that is currently used for the manufacture of most root canal instruments is 56 m% Ni and 44 m% Ti. These proportions are used because even a 2% change in the metal composition can dramatically change the mechanical properties of the material, especially hardness and elasticity. NiTi endodontic instruments for both manual and power-driven root canal instrumentation are available worldwide from numerous manufacturers.

Case Presentation

A Radiographic diagnosis of a mandibular molar.

B An NiTi Sensor File is used in the canal following coronal expansion with Gates drills.

C NiTi files cannot be prebent. They are used at a speed of ca. 250 rpm.

D The files are characterized by extraordinary flexibility.

E Following a radiographic measurement, the apical segment is treated using files with 2% conicity.

F Radiograph of the completed endodontic therapy.

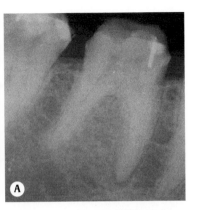

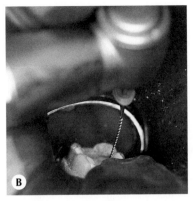

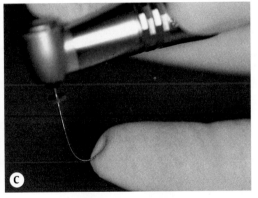

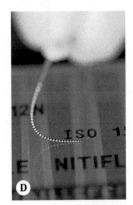

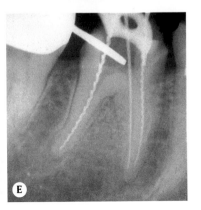

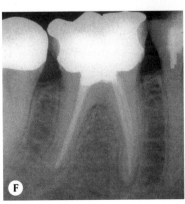

The Lightspeed (LS) set consists of 22 instruments. The **instrument tip** is similar to a Gates-Glidden drill and consists of two parts: the noncutting **pilot tip** and a cutting portion. The cutting portion is 0.25–1.75 mm long, depending upon instrument size. The head geometry varies according to instrument size: With increasing size, the instrument heads are also larger. The **shaft** of LS instruments is thinner than the cutting head, and very flexible. It is not conical; with increasing instrument size the diameter of the shaft also increases, but not as much as with conventional instruments. For example, the shaft of a size 80 instrument has a diameter of 0.50 mm.

Following trepanation, instrumentation of the root canal begins analogous to the step-down technique, with conventional **Gates-Glidden** drills. The Gates drill size 1 (#50) is used to widen the canal up to any dilaceration at a speed of 500 rpm, and the instrument tip is coated with a lubricant. The size 2 Gates drill (#70) is adjusted 1 mm shorter, size 3 is set 2 mm shorter, and #4 and #5 are also adjusted accordingly shorter.

Following coronal expansion, the working length is radiographically determined using a size 15 K file. If the K file cannot be inserted to the working length because of a very narrow root canal, a Hedström file must be carefully used to establish patency to the working length. Subsequently, another radiograph is taken to confirm the working length/depth.

Instead of the step-down technique, one may elect to begin using the crown-down technique coronally. This involves first the use of a #5 Gates drill to widen the orifice, and then smaller Gates drills are used to penetrate ever more deeply into the canal.

Following radiographic determination of the working length, a K file #15 is used to instrument the root canal to the full working length. Lightspeed instruments are available at only size 20 and above, therefore the initial entrance to the working length must always be performed manually with a #15 file.

Following copious rinsing of the canal with sodium hypochlorite solution, a size 20 **Lightspeed** instrument is inserted into the canal to the working length, using a lubricant. The speed is set at 900 rpm. The initial goal is to prepare an apical stop. Next, a size 22.5 is ad-

justed to the same length, followed by reinsertion of the #15 K file. Following Lightspeed file size 22.5, sizes 25, 27.5, and 30 etc. are utilized. The first LS instrument that binds in the root canal at full working length is called the **"initial apical rotatory"** or IAR. It is recommended that, following IAR, the root canal should be instrumented to full length, five additional instrument sizes, usually to size 40.

Using LS instruments, it is necessary to employ a careful insertion and a definitive withdrawal movement in order to remove all dentinal debris from the canal. Each file is used only once in the canal, and after each file copious canal rinsing is imperative.

The final instrument with which the apical stop is prepared is termed the **"master apical rotary"** or MAR. This is followed by a step-back preparation. During this procedure, each additional LS instrument is shortened by 1 mm from the established working length. Depending upon the canal length, this is continued until the achievement of the final step-down procedure. This technique provides a uniformly conical canal shape.

Case Presentation

A Diagnostic radiograph of a maxillary premolar.

B Coronal widening using Gates-Glidden drills according to the step-down technique.

C Using small Gates drills, one penetrates deeper until reaching any dilaceration.

D Coronal widening with Gates drills follows length determination and apical expansion with a #15 K file. Additional apical widening is performed using four additional instrument sizes, and a conical shape is prepared via the step-back technique.

E The apical preparation is performed using small Lightspeed instruments.

F Following instrumentation to the MAR, all subsequent instruments are adjusted appropriately shorter.

G Final radiograph clearly shows the conical shape of the preparation.

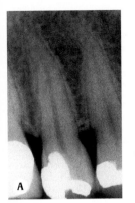

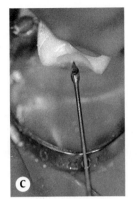

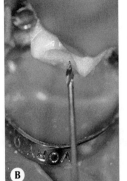

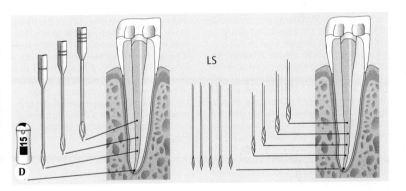

LS

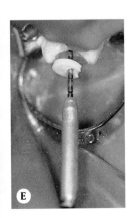

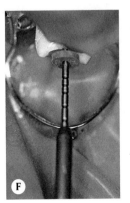

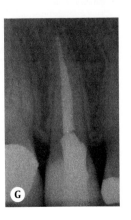

Quantec instruments exhibit wide lateral radial lands behind sharp cutting edges. According to the manufacturer, the positive cutting angle cuts dentin more effectively, and the design of the between-edge spaces permits improved removal of dentin chips and debris. The LX version has a noncutting tip, which guides the instrument better into dilacerated canals.

Ten Quantec instruments are commercially available. Instrument #1 exhibits a 6% conicity and is only 17mm long. The instrument tip corresponds to size 25. Instruments #2–4 all exhibit a 2% conicity and correspond to sizes 15, 20, and 25. Instruments #5–8 are differentiated by identical size (#25) but a 3–6% increasing conicity. Instrument #9 has a 2% increase corresponding to size 40, and #10 to size 45. Most recently, three additional instruments have become available with concities 8, 10, and 12%; these are indicated for additional conical shaping of the root canal.

Following a brief phase of expansion, Quantec files are immediately used to the full working length. **Coronal widening** is performed with file #1. After determining the working length, file #2 is used to instrument the canal to its **full length** up to size 15, #3 up to size 20 and #3 to size 25. This series completes the **apical instrumentation**.

The next four files are used for conical **shaping**. Because the next files all are of size 25, but have increasing conicity (3, 4, 5, and 6%), the final canal preparation results in a satisfactory conical shape.

Using a second instrumentation sequence, the files with 12% conicity can be used following initial instrumentation with file #1 (17mm long, 6% conicity). One subsequently uses the files with 10% conicity, which penetrate deeper into the canal. The files with 8% conicity proceed still deeper, and the 6% conicity file reaches any canal dilaceration without difficulty. Only at this point is the working length determined radiographically, and files #2–4 used to the full working length.

In a third variation, all of the Quantec files can be used in the crown-down technique by starting with a 12% conicity file coronally and then with smaller conicity files deeper and deeper into the root canal. This is performed in several sequences until files with 3% conic-

ity almost reach to the apical foramen, and finally file size 25 (with 2% conicity) extends to the apical constriction. In this technique, no files of size 15 and 20 with 2% conicity are employed.

In comparative studies, the Quantec system resulted in somewhat poorer canal shaping vis-à-vis the HERO 642 system. Using simulated plastic root canals, a good canal shape with uniform conicity was achieved. In canals with more severe dilaceration, perforations occurred and also pronounced expansion on the external curvature of the canal. In studies of cleansing efficacy, no differences were noted between the Quantec and Lightspeed instruments. Cleansing by both systems was uniform and characterized as "good." An analysis of 378 Quantec instruments that had been used under dental practice conditions revealed obvious defects on 50% of the instruments; 21% exhibited signs of torsion fractures and bending fractures, 28% also showed other deformations. It was speculated that the most important cause of fracture was excessive apically directed force during instrumentation. Although the amount of torque required to induce a fracture was well above the amount of torque during actual instrumentation, the range and standard deviations were enormous.

Case Presentation

A Diagnostic radiograph of a mandibular molar.

B Coronal opening with the 17mm long instrument exhibiting 6% conicity.

C Determining the working length.

D/E Schematic of the procedure: Opening into the middle third of the canal, subsequent apical widening, and further conical shaping to the full length.

F Apical widening to size 25.

G Shaping, with increasing conicity.

H Radiograph of the root canal fillings exhibits the conical canal preparations.

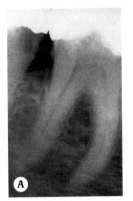

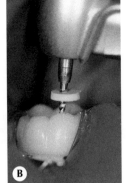

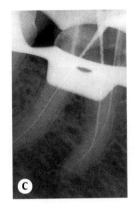

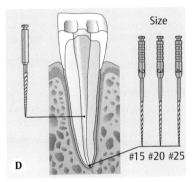

Size

#15 #20 #25

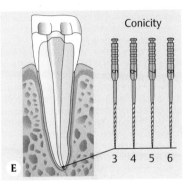

Conicity

3 4 5 6

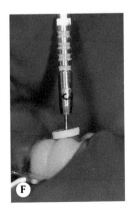

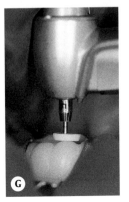

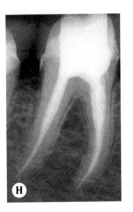

One of the first **NiTi systems** was the ProFile instruments, which have proved themselves in daily practice for many years. The instrument set consists of orifice shapers (19 mm long files with 5–8% conicity), the conical ProFile 06 with a 6% conicity in sizes 15–40, as well as the ProFile 04 with a conicity of 4% in sizes 15–90. Orifice shapers are used for instrumentation of the coronal third of the root canal. The ProFile 06 instrument with a length 21 or 25 mm is used for instrumentation of the middle third. Instrumentation of the apical segment is accomplished with the ProFile 04 files (lengths 21, 25, and 31 mm).

The instruments have a U-shaped cross-sectional profile and "**radial lands.**" These maintain the instruments centered within the canal, and permit easy smoothing of the canal walls. They prevent any binding or catching/sticking in dentin. The smooth, noncutting tip serves to guide the file within the canal without scratching or gouging.

In a comparative study between and among ProFile, Flexofile, and the KaVo-Endo system, 120 extracted teeth were instrumented; 60 had straight roots and 60 exhibited at least one dilacerated root. It was demonstrated that the ProFile system instruments did not cause any alteration in the form or the course of the canals. However, the cleansing efficiency of the ProFile system was less than with manual instrumentation.

After rinsing with EDTA, files from the ProFile series provided the cleanest canal walls; after rinsing with sodium hypochlorite, the ProFile system gave poorer results.

When using the **crown-down instrumentation technique**, one uses two instruments in two different sizes (colors):

- for **wide root canals**, one begins with the blue Orifice Shapers to expand coronally
- subsequently, a red Orifice Shaper extends deeper into the coronal segment of the canal
- then a blue ProFile 06 is used, and thereafter a red ProFile 06, which should penetrate into the apical third of the root canal
- at this point, the working length is determined radiographically
- the yellow ProFile 04 widens and instruments the root canal to its full length, followed by the red and the blue ProFile 04.

For **average size canals**, one begins with a red Orifice Shaper, penetrates more deeply with a yellow instrument, followed by a red and a yellow ProFile 06. The final apical instrumentation, following working length determination, is performed first with a yellow ProFile 04 to full canal length, followed by red and blue.

The ProFile instruments must always be coated with a lubricant, and between each change of instruments the canal must be copiously rinsed with 5% NaOCl solution.

The ProFile instruments are used with a slight **in-and-out movement**, with a hub motion of not more than 2 mm and with only slight application of force.

ProFile instruments can only be used in combination with a motor that has torsion limiter (e.g., ATR Technica), with low rpm (250–350). This will prevent over-twisting the instrument and resultant fracture.

No ProFile instrument should be used more than 10 times.

Case Presentation

A One begins the coronal opening with a blue Orifice Shaper; then a red Orifice Shaper is used up into the middle third of the root canal. A blue ProFile 06 extends deeper into the canal, followed by the red ProFile 06.

B After instrumentation of the coronal segment of the root canal, a blue and then a red ProFile 04 are employed. When a point has been reached about 2–3 mm short of the apical constriction, working length is determined, and then the preparation is completed to full working length with ProFile 04 instruments from yellow through blue.

C Initiating the instrumentation with a blue Orifice Shaper ...

D ... followed by the red instrument.

E The ProFile 06 penetrates into the apical third.

F The ProFile 04 is used to instrument the entire canal length.

G Conclusion using a blue ProFile 04.

H Final radiograph depicting the clinical result.

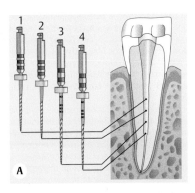

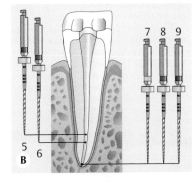

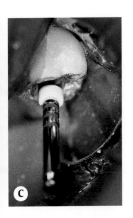

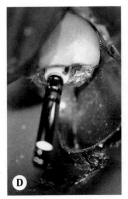

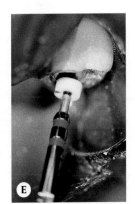

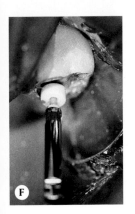

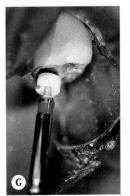

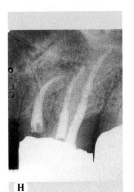

The original **Greater-Taper** or GT Rotary instrument set derives from Buchanan (1996), and is available commercially from the Tulsa Dental Company, mainly for the American market. It consists of six instruments (GT Rotary files 06 #20, 08 #20, 10 #20 as well as GT accessory files 12 #35, 12 #50, and 12 #70). In Europe, these instruments are manufactured by the Swiss firm Maillefer, and have been expanded by four additional instruments of the ProFile systems 04: 04 #20, 04 #25, 04 #30, and 04 #35.

The GT files are instruments with identical **size**, but differing **conicity**.

Recently this system (NiTi-GT "new") has been expanded by two file sequences: For small root canals, files in size 30 are available, and in wide canals files up to size 40. The conicity is 4, 6, 8, and 10%, and even 12% with the accessory files.

A characteristic of the GT Rotary set is the high conicity, which is designed to provide a conical shape of the entire root canal during root canal instrumentation, including a broad coronal opening.

With all GT-Rotary files, the angle of attack is neutral. The tips are smooth and noncutting. The angle of the cutting edge to the long axis increases from the instrument tip up to the end of the working portion in the ProFile instruments and the accessory files. With the GT files, it is same on all segments of the working portion, at ca. 30°.

The files are designed for use at 250–300 rpm, except those with a conicity of 12%, which can be used at up to 500 rpm because of their larger diameter. Instrumentation is performed using the crown-down technique.

The initial widening of the canal orifices using accessory file #35 or #50 depending upon the size of the canal is followed by the actual root canal instrumentation with files of 10% conicity increasing up to 6% conicity. Apical instrumentation is performed exclusively using files of 4% conicity. Using the #10 file, the entire coronal segment is instrumented; the #8 penetrates several mm deeper into the canal, and the #6 file achieves the canal apex.

In a second sequence, the #8 file is again used, but now it penetrates to the same depth as the previous #6 file had achieved. Subsequently, the #6 file penetrates to shortly before the apical constriction.

Following precise radiographic determination of the **working depth**, the 04 file is used at the working length. In contrast to the crown-down technique, the files with 4% conicity are used from small through large, i.e., size 20 is used first to the working length. Thereafter, sizes 25 and 30 are employed to the same depth.

The selection of files is dependent upon the size and degree of dilaceration of the root canal (one differentiates only between small and large). The smaller the root, the smaller should be the size of the instruments utilized. The more severe the root canal dilaceration, the smaller the conicity of instruments used in the apical segment.

Case Presentation

A One begins the coronal widening of the canal orifice with a file exhibiting 12% conicity. Files with 10% conicity penetrate deeper into the canal, those with 8% conicity achieve the middle third of the canal, and files with 6% conicity finally extend into the apical third.

B After determination of the working length, files with 4% conicity are used with increasing size 20–30 to the full working length.

C Coronal expansion using 12% conicity.

D Deep penetration with lesser conicities.

E Working length determination in the radiograph.

F Apical instrumentation beginning with #20.

G Completing the instrumentation with size 30.

H Final radiograph after endodontic treatment.

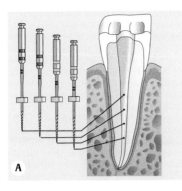

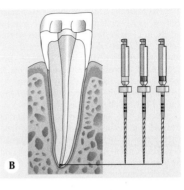

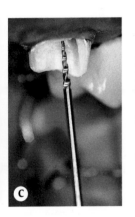

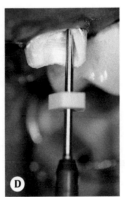

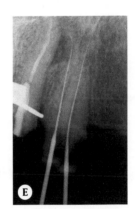

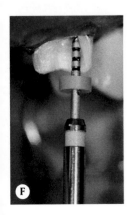

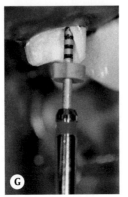

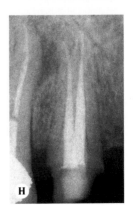

The FlexMaster system exhibits a **triangular convex cross-section**, with sharp cutting edges. In contrast to other NiTi systems, the FlexMaster's massive instrument core should guarantee reduced danger of breakage because of an increased resistance to torsion, at least in straight root canals. For efficient instrumentation, the convex cutting surfaces and the cutting edges of the type K file are incorporated. FlexMaster does not incorporate the wide radial lands of previously described NiTi systems, which provided, above all, good centering. Speeds of 150 and 300rpm should be used with these power-driven files.

The instrument set is provided in a convenient box; the files are clearly arranged, and therefore ensure efficient and simplified clinical use. The set consists of a short, highly conical Interofile for coronal instrumentation, also three files with 4–6% conicity in sizes 20, 25 and 30, as well as files with 2% conicity in sizes 20–35. Additional sizes can be ordered.

Instrumentation is performed using the crown-down technique. Working with the FlexMaster requires:
• large, straight access cavity
• determination of the working length following coronal instrumentation
• maintaining constant rpm
• gentle up and down movement of the instrument, without excessive forcing apically.

Individual instrument use should be limited to a maximum of 10 seconds. Instruments are inserted into the moist canal with a lubricant. The number of uses must be documented, and must not exceed eight. Constant optical control during clinical procedures should involve magnifying loupes to detect and discard any instruments that are deformed and therefore susceptible to fracture.

Instrumentation is divided into a **crown-down** sequence and an **apical sequence**. Instrumentation of the coronal root canal segment is performed with files of 4 and 6% conicity; apical preparation employs files with 2% conicity. Within the sequence of use, one differentiates among the instrumentation of wide, average and narrow root canals (blue, red, and yellow sequence).

Before each crown-down step, first the Interofile is used to widen the canal orifices as well as the first 10–12mm, in some cases up to any canal dilaceration. The blue sequence begins with the blue file 06/30 (conicity 6%, size 30); the red file 06/25 penetrates somewhat deeper into the canal, followed by the yellow file 06/20. The final instrument used in this sequence is blue file 04/30; it penetrates beyond any canal dilacerations, extending into the apical region of the canal. If the region 2–3mm before the apical constriction is not achieved, the crown-down sequence is again completely performed. If this point is already achieved with the second or third file, the coronal instrumentation is complete and the radiographic determination of **working length** is performed.

For instrumentation of the apical portion of the canal, one uses exclusively files with 2% conicity, because in dilacerated canals they are extraordinarily flexible and therefore considerably less susceptible to fracture. One initiates the instrumentation with size 20 and, depending upon the size of the root canal, concludes with size 30 or higher.

Case Presentation

A Diagnostic radiograph

B Initiating the coronal instrumentation with the red sequence (06/25) in an average size canal. Lengths on these instruments are engraved on the shaft (18, 19, 20, and 22mm), so that during the first phase of instrumentation the clinician can work without the rubber reference stop.

C Deeper insertion with the second file 06/20.

D The blue crown-down sequence in large diameter root canals begins with 06/30, and ends with 04/30.

E Apical instrumentation using files with 2% conicity, beginning with 02/20.

F Third step of the crown-down sequence. The 2-mm point has already been reached.

G Apical instrumentation beginning with 02/20.

H Final radiograph of the filled canals.

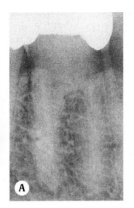

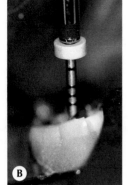

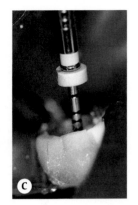

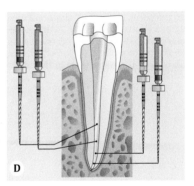

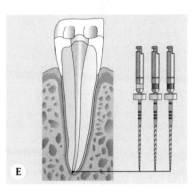

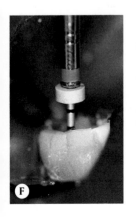

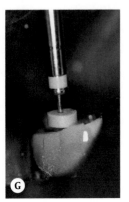

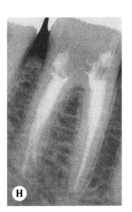

The K3 endodontic instruments are NiTi files of ISO sizes 15–60, with conicities of 4, 6, 8, and 10%. Files with 8% or 10% conicity serve as initial canal orifice wideners.

A special characteristic of the instruments is their **asymmetric cross-sectional profile**. The cutting surfaces of the instruments exhibit a positive angle of attack.

The **angle of attack** indicates the angle of the cutting surfaces to the access of rotation, and also indicates how materials are removed during root canal instrumentation. One differentiates among neutral, positive, and negative angle of attack:

- with a positive angle of attack, the cutting is performed in the same direction as the applied force, and is active
- with a neutral angle of attack, the cutting is perpendicular to the canal wall
- a nonactive cutting effect occurs with a negative angle of attack.

On average, the cutting efficiency of the K3 files is greater than the GT-Rotary. The level of cutting efficiency is probably determined for the most part by the shape and form of the cutting edges.

A study by Stelzner (2003) was unable to corroborate the manufacturer's statements concerning the effect of a positive cutting angle on the efficiency on the K3 instruments. While it **was** found that the K3 files on average cut more deeply than instruments from the GT-Rotary group, the differences were not statistically significant. In this study, instruments from the GT-Rotary group and the K3 group exhibited the lowest cutting efficiency.

In addition to the ProTaper instruments, the FlexMaster files achieved the highest cutting efficiency. With these instruments, the cutting efficiency increased with increasing instrument size. One common characteristic of the FlexMaster and ProTaper instruments, which appear to have higher cutting efficiencies in comparison to the K3 and GT-Rotary files, is their similar cross-sectional profile: both exhibit a triangular instrument cross-section, with pointed cutting edges and convex cutting surfaces.

The removal of dentin from the root canal wall is therefore more difficult because the edges of the K3 files are not capable of cutting effectively into the dentin. The "cutting efficiency" in this case is more an effect of abrasion. The addition of a concave profile of the cutting surfaces, as with the GT-Rotary files, reduces the angle of attack and therefore reduces the cutting efficiency. Due to the relatively large contact surface of the instrument with the canal wall in files with "radial land," the frictional resistance is increased and this also elevates the danger of instrument fracture.

Instrumentation should be performed at 250–300 rpm.

After taking a diagnostic initial radiograph, the files for the orifice widening (10 #25 or 08 #25) are used to instrument down to any canal dilaceration. Then, after radiographic measurement, instruments with a conicity of 6% in decreasing sizes 35, 30, 25, 20 are used to achieve the working length. For narrow and dilacerated root canals, the use of files with 4% conicity is recommended in the dilacerated region.

Case Presentation

A Coronal instrumentation begins with a file exhibiting 10% conicity. A #8 file penetrates to the middle portion of the canal, and the #6 file to the transition in the apical third of the canal. All three instruments correspond to size 25 at the apex.

B The canal is instrumented to the working length with #4 files in ascending sizes.

C/D Coronal opening of the root canals in the crown-down technique using files exhibiting 6–10% conicity.

E Radiographic length determination

F/G Apical instrumentation with 4% conicity.

H Final radiograph.

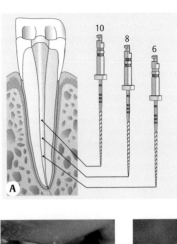

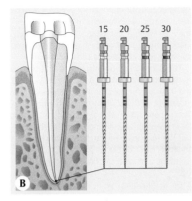

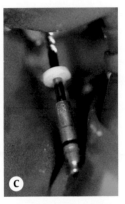

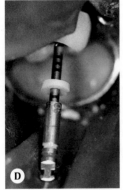

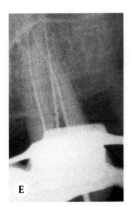

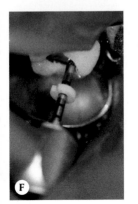

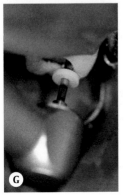

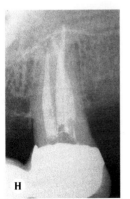

ProTaper instruments have a very unconventional shape; they combine in a single file several **(ascending) conicities**. There are three shaping files for coronal expansion and three finishing files for shaping the apical region.

The diameter of the instruments at the tip of the working portion is between 0.17/0.19 and 0.20 mm for the shaping files, while these values are 0.20/0.25/0.30 mm for the finishing files. In contrast to other types of instruments, the ProTaper files exhibit conicities between 2 and 19% in a single file. In the **shaping files**, the gradient toward the instrument tip is descending, and with the **finishing files** ascending.

Up to finishing file 3, all instruments exhibit a triangular cross-sectional profile with convex cutting edges. The cross-section of file F3 is characterized by a modified triangular form with concave surfaces, but does not otherwise differ significantly from the other files. All instruments exhibit a rounded, noncutting tip; the cutting edges of the working area extend almost to the tip. Because of the changing conicities, the tangent angle varies considerably, between 20 and 30°. However, in all instruments it **increases** from the instrument tip to the coronal end of the working portion.

Canal instrumentation begins with shaping file #1, which simultaneously widens more aggressively at the coronal aspect but which can already be inserted to the working length. Next, shaping file #2 (under electronic length control) is used to instrument to the apex, and the **working length** is precisely determined radiographically. Now one can begin with finishing file size 20 to instrument and widen the root canal along its entire length, and to instrument apically further up to sizes 25 and 30.

In contrast to the other two nitinol instrument types, ProTaper instruments have the important advantage that even during initial instrumentation of the coronal root canal segments, widening up to the size of the corresponding Gates-Glidden drills 4–5 (sizes 110–130) can be achieved; this simplifies significantly further apical instrumentation, as well as the subsequent filling of the canal via gutta percha condensation.

The files are inserted into the canal using gentle in-and-out movements with amplitude of about 1 mm; the files must be cleaned frequently, because during initial instrumentation large amounts of dentin are removed. The removed dentin can accumulate between the cutting edges and may lead to wedging of the file within the canal. Cleaning with sterile gauze and frequent rinsing of the canal with NaOCl are necessary.

Because instruments F2 and F3 fracture significantly easier in severely dilacerated root canals in comparison to files of lesser conicity, in these cases one should combine coronal instrumentation with shaping files and the apical instrumentation using Profile 04 or Flex-Master 04, or in extremely dilacerated canals even the FlexMaster 02.

Cleansing of the root canal surface by instruments with a U-shaped cross-section and "radial lands" (ProFile, GT-Rotary) provides better results when compared with the Flex-Master and ProTaper systems with conventional triangular cross-section. The U-shaped cross-section evacuates dentin chips more effectively and, in addition, the improved centering of the instruments provides efficient cleansing, without creating pouch-like expansion at the critical apical region.

Case Presentation

A Instrument sequence in straight root canals: coronal instrumentation with S1 and S1 is followed by apical shaping with F1–F3.

B In dilacerated root canals, apical instrumentation is performed with ProFile 04, sizes 20–30.

C Initial entry preparation using the SX file.

D The tip is coated with a lubricant.

E Coronal instrumentation using the S1 file.

F Finishing files are used for instrumentation in the apical segment.

G The F3 files is used to instrument straight sections of the root canal.

H Final radiograph of the filled root canals.

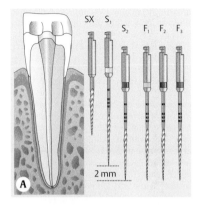

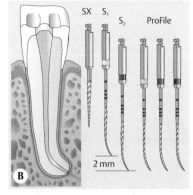

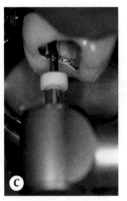

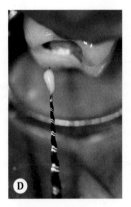

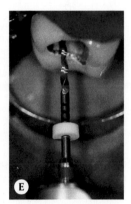

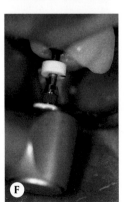

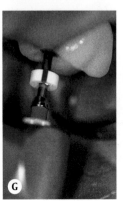

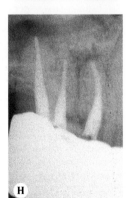

Straight root canals instrumented manually or with sonic or ultrasonic files can be instrumented completely during the first appointment. On the other hand, **dilacerated canals** will not be completely freed of infected pulpal tissue debris, regardless of the technique employed. As a result, it becomes clear that **root canal anatomy** influences the resulting effectiveness of canal instrumentation more than any special instrumentation technique.

Proper and thorough instrumentation of the root canal is the very basis for a successful root canal filling.

In an SEM study, neither the nickel-titanium systems ProFile, GT-Rotary, FlexMaster nor ProTaper achieved complete cleansing of dilacerated root canals. With regard to removal of debris, the instruments with a U-shaped cross-section (ProFile, GT-Rotary) provided better results than those with a triangular cross-section (FlexMaster, ProTaper). Statistical evaluation of the comparison among systems revealed significant differences in the amount of debris accumulation in the apical root canal segment.

Several investigations have demonstrated that manual instrumentation results in a more effective cleansing of the canal, with adequate removal of dentin debris, when compared with power-driven systems.

A mostly homogeneous "smear layer" upon the entire root canal wall exists after instrumentation using all of the systems described. ProTaper files, GT-Rotary, and manual instrumentation result in a thin smear layer in some areas. Instrumenting with GT-Rotary files results in a thicker smear layer, especially apically, and with blockage of the adjacent dentinal tubuli.

With EDTA and sodium hypochlorite rinsing, ProFile instruments leave behind a less pronounced smear layer. Irrigation with EDTA solution dissolves this smear layer.

The **smear layer** is created upon the canal wall surfaces as a result of instrumentation, and leads to closure of the dentinal tubuli orifices. Even canal instrumentation using sonic and ultrasonic devices cannot prevent the formation of a smear layer. One differentiates between the dentin debris forced into the dentinal tubuli and the smear layer that accumulates on the root canal walls. Electron

microscopic examination provided no clear differentiation between the smear layer and other root dentin.

The smear layer creates a diffusion barrier that reduces the permeability of dentin by 25–30%. If the smear layer is removed, root canal dressings containing medicaments can better diffuse into the dentin of the canal walls, and the antibacterial effect increases. The use of EDTA as the final rinsing solution completely removes the smear layer; in addition, the dentinal tubuli orifices become larger because of the dissolution of peritubular dentin. Bacteria readily adhere to the smear layer. The removal of this layer by means of citric acid followed by NaOCl solution causes about a 15% higher freedom from bacteria on the simultaneously clean root canal surfaces.

Importantly, however, dissolution of the smear layer by chelators and acids also brings with it certain dangers. In an invitro experiment on extracted teeth, removal of the smear layer with citric acid led, three weeks after inoculation of the root canals, to deep bacterial penetration into the adjacent dentinal tubuli (*S. faecium*). In the control group with an intact smear layer, bacteria were only observed on the dentin surface. The conclusion is that an intact smear layer renders the attachment and penetration of bacteria more difficult.

Illustrations

A–C Following instrumentation of the apical segment of the root canal, one notes an irregular canal surface with dentin accumulations that indicate insufficient tissue removal. At higher magnification, one clearly notes an even smear layer with large accumulations of soft tissue debris.

D/E The middle third of the canal is well cleansed and free of any larger tissue debris accumulations. Higher magnification reveals the almost completely closure of dentinal tubuli by an even smear layer.

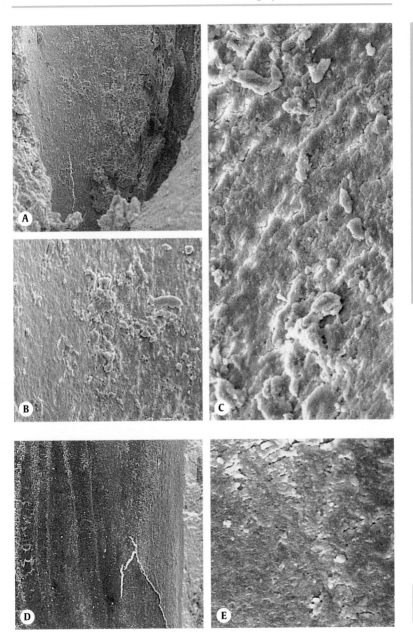

In the early days of power-driven root canal instrumentation, the frequent incidence of **instrument fracture** represented a serious problem. The majority of fractures occurred when the instrument wedged within the canal and the subsequent forces exceeded the **torsion** limit, which for each instrument is especially dependent on canal dilaceration and the radius of the flexure. Instruments can resist elastic deformation, but only over a small range. Following the initial elastic deformation, instrument fracture can occur relatively quickly, usually without previous deformation of the cutting edges.

In straight root canals, fracture is a function of the instrument size and its conicity; larger instruments and those with larger conicity fracture later. In **dilacerated canals**, the occurrence of instrument fracture follows a different set of rules: Here, the smaller **conicities** are maximally loaded; the greater the conicity, the earlier will instrument fracture occur. Instrument-loading resistance is also dependent on the radius of the apical curvature. With a large radius of curvature, instruments fracture significantly later than with a small radius; the curvature angle appears to play a less significant role. Speed also influences instrument fracture; if speed is reduced from 300 to 150 rpm, the danger of fracture is lower.

A micromotor developed especially for the use of NiTi files should **exclude** the risk of instrument fracture.

Illustrations

A *TCM Endo (Nouvag AG):*
This motor has selectable torque and rpm speed, and is, with few exceptions, indicated for all NiTi systems. When one of the five selected torques is reached (2), the motor switches into reverse. However, precise numbers for torque or torsion are not provided.

B *Endostepper (SET):*
The computer chip-controlled step motor completes 1600 individual steps per revolution. When the critical moment of torque is reached, the motor stops immediately. Using a foot pedal, the file can then be rotated left or right-left and removed from the canal. Button F1 choses the appropriate file, and F2 selects the file sequence.

C *ATR Technika (ATR Pistoia):*
The ATR motor is programmable for all systems. Using the system button, the file system is selected, and with the program button, the files to be employed. Torque and speed (rpm) can be adapted freely to the clinical situation. Two speed buttons, T_{min} and T_{max}, reduce or increase the programmed torque value by 25%, and are selected for either straight or dilacerated canals. The factory-set adjustments are usually only usable for mildly dilacerated canals.

D *ATR Technika Vision:*
This further development of the ATR motor contains two program cards on which the individually changed settings are programmed. This should permit more dentists to use this motor with their own Smart Cards.

E *E-Master (VDW):*
This is a smaller and much lighter motor, which can only be used with FlexMaster files. The display corresponds to the arrangement of the system box, in which the files are sorted such that they can be used for large, average, or narrow canals. If the load upon the instrument exceeds the expected torque value, the motor changes direction. The motor is also easily mounted on the bracket table.

F *Endo IT control (VDW):*
This motor provides individual torque programming: When the torque limit is reached, the motor automatically changes direction. When 75% of the programmed value is achieved, an audible warning signal is provided. Within the "file library" all contemporary endodontic file systems are programmed with two separate levels, one for novices and another for experienced clinicians. Torque as well as speed can be changed and adapted to individual canal anatomy/geometry. However, if a new file is inserted, the factory-set adjustment is automatically programmed (in contrast to the ATR motor).

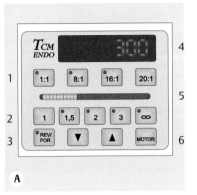

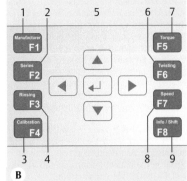

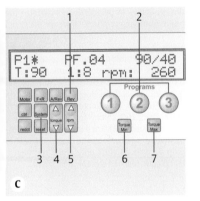

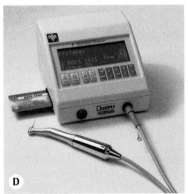

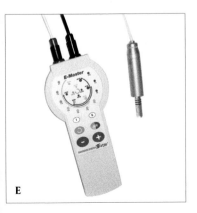

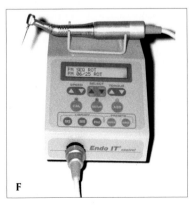

Numerous scientific studies have demonstrated that it is not possible to achieve a **sterile** root canal even after thorough cleansing, instrumentation, and rinsing. This fact has led to long discussions concerning microorganisms left behind in the root canal, and the possible consequences. It has been demonstrated that bacteria rapidly proliferate within a root canal if it is not filled or treated with a disinfectant dressing between two appointments.

Bacteria have been identified within necrotic pulpal tissues, on the root canal surface and within dentinal tubuli. In cases of apical periodontitis, bacteria are always detectable within the endodontium.

Periapical lesions present a **mixed infection** consisting of two to 12 bacterial species. There exists a direct correlation between the size of the apical lesions and the number of bacteria in the root canal. On the other hand, following failed endodontic treatment, only one or two bacterial species dominate, especially gram-positive microorganisms. **Enterococcus faecalis** is the single most predominant bacterial component.

Initially occurring periapical lesions with clinical symptoms are almost always accompanied by the presence of certain microbes within the endodontium. *Prevotella buccae, Porphyromonas endodontalis*, as well as *Porphyromonas gingivalis*, are always present in teeth with pain, percussion sensitivity, and intraoral fistula. Studies have also shown a relationship between black-pigmenting bacteria and clinically acute lesions with spontaneous pain. Identification and presence of these microorganisms has also been associated with persistent pain following endodontic therapy.

Bacteria are not found **only** on the root canal surfaces or within infected and necrotic pulpal tissues. Viable bacteria have also been demonstrated in specimens of dentin taken 0.5–2 mm distant from the root canal surface. Histologic studies have even demonstrated bacteria that had penetrated half the distance to the dentin-cementum junction.

Endotoxin is also routinely detected **within** the dentin of an infected root canal.

Experimental studies have shown that if dentin adjacent to the root canal pulp is inoculated with bacteria, these microbes penetrate the adjacent dentinal tubuli and remain viable for up to ten days.

Certain factors appear to influence the depth of bacterial penetration: Before the smear layer created by instrumentation of the root canal is dissolved and removed by **citric acid** or **EDTA solution**, no penetration of bacteria occurs.

Enterococcus faecalis and *Streptococcus sanguis* penetrate into the dentinal tubuli up to a depth of 400 µm within two weeks, while *Pseudomonas aeruginosa* and *Bacteroides melaninogenicus* don't penetrate the tubuli even after four weeks of incubation. Bacteria within the pulp penetrate deeper into dentin if the cementum covering the root surface is removed. If the root surface is exposed and no longer covered by cementum, bacteria have the capability to penetrate and colonize the tubuli from the periphery. However, the speed of penetration from the external approach is lower.

In teeth exhibiting moderate to severe periodontitis, with deep pocket formation, bacteria will exist on the external root surface and represent a potential danger to the pulp. In caries-free but periodontally involved teeth, more than 100 colony-forming units were demonstrated in 27 % of dentin specimens immediately adjacent to the pulp. The entire pulp became necrotic only when the microbial plaque reached the apical foramen.

Illustrations

A In the presence of a smear layer, bacteria on the pulpal aspect of the dentin surface are incapable of penetrating dentinal tubuli. However, if the smear layer is removed, certain bacteria can penetrate.

B Cross-sectional microscopic view of dentinal tubuli with bacteria.

C Longer term bacterial demineralization in coronal root canal sections.

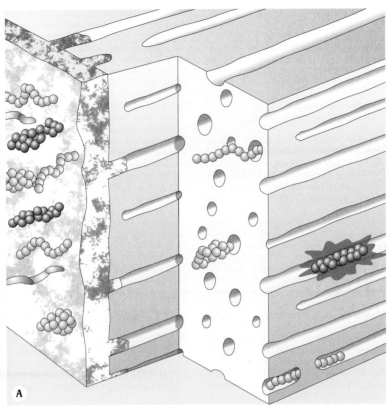

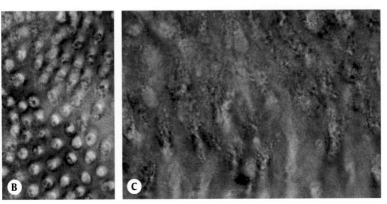

Canal rinsing should:
• float dentin chips out of the canal, therefore preventing blockage
• dissolve vital and also necrotic tissue debris in those areas not accessible for manual instrumentation
• provide a lubrication effect for the instruments
• have an antibacterial effect
• have some bleaching effect.

The active ingredient in a rinsing solution should have the highest possible antibacterial effect, but low tissue toxicity.

Still today, the most important rinsing solution is **sodium hypochlorite**. This was used very early on in a modified form by Semmelweis as a hand disinfection agent. NaOCl solution is colorless to green/yellow and has a mild odor of chlorine; the pH value is between 10.7 and 12.2. It is unstable to light and heat. In a study of teeth that were autoclaved and then incubated with various microorganisms, sodium hypochlorite reduced the bacterial number. When compared with a 0.5% solution, the antibacterial activity of a 2.5% solution was 3.5× higher, and that of a 5.25% solution 5.5× higher.

The dissolution of necrotic pulpal tissue is one most important properties of a rinsing solution. In a test of cleansing effectiveness, instrumented root canals exhibited a cleaner surface after rinsing with a 2% NaOCl solution. Even in the first 15 minutes after rinsing with a 2% NaOCl solution, 15% of the pulpal soft tissues were dissolved; after 60 minutes, 45% and after two hours all pulpal tissue was dissolved. This underscores the significance of treatment duration. The higher the NaOCl concentration, the faster the dissolution. With a 6% solution, 98% of the canal surface was clean and free of tissue debris after 20 minutes. The recommended maximum concentration is 5.25%, however, because increasing beyond this level is associated with increased tissue toxicity.

Hydrogen peroxide (H_2O_2) removes tissue debris and dentin chips from the canal, but its tissue-dissolving capability is very low. The recommendation is a 3% solution. Because endodontic lubricants contain peroxide, additional rinsing may be avoidable.

As a chelate builder or chelator, **EDTA solution** (ethylendiamine tetra-acetate) effectively binds divalent ions. It has a pH value of 7.3, but has a relatively low antibacterial effect. At a 10–15% concentration, however, it is very effective in dissolving tissue debris and the smear layer. Therefore, like **citric-acid rinsing**, EDTA solution is recommended before the placement of calcium hydroxide. At a 15% concentration, citric acid has been shown to be very effective against anaerobic bacteria.

Solvidont, a bisdequalium acetate, exhibits good antibacterial properties, but also an unfavorable relationship between cytotoxicity and antibacterial efficiency.

Physiologic saline (NaCl) is by far the most tissue-friendly rinsing solution, but its antibacterial effect is quite low.

Iodine and also potassium iodide are good antiseptics with equally good tissue biocompatibility. "Betadine" is the commercially available product.

With **paraformaldehyde** or **phenol-containing solutions**, on the other hand, the tissue toxicity is higher than the antibacterial efficacy.

Case Presentation

A Rinsing cannulae should screw securely onto the disposable syringe.

B The thin cannulae must be evenly bent and must not be kinked. The device for bending files (Endobent) can also be used for cannulae.

C The canal should be thoroughly rinsed between each change of files. Every root canal should be rinsed with at least 20 mL of NaOCl.

D For an effective antibacterial and tissue dissolving effect, it is important that the rinsing cannula penetrate deeply into the canal. This is virtually guaranteed when using the crown-down technique.

E/F The smallest rinsing cannula has a diameter of 0.35 mm and therefore can follow the last Gates-Glidden drill up to the canal dilaceration.

G/H Root canal instrumentation using 5% NaOCl and citric acid rinsing solutions.

I Radiograph appearance two years later.

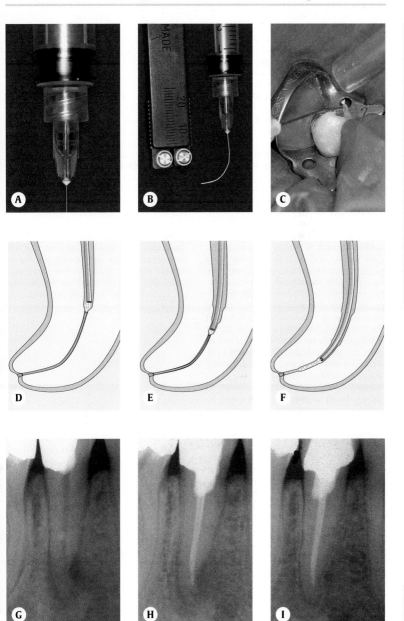

The effect and efficiency of root-canal rinsing can be increased through the simultaneous use of **ultrasonic files**. This is attributed to several factors:

- the high frequency vibrations of the file transport the sodium hypochlorite rinsing solution effectively into the apical regions of the canal
- the liquid within the canal is mixed better and the solution is warmed.

The ultrasonic frequencies of the devices lie between 25 and 40 kHz. During actual instrumentation, the energy is mainly disengaged **longitudinally**, and only a small portion is transformed into **transverse vibrations**. Even a small load prevents the oscillation.

Important ultrasonic phenomena are cavitation and so-called "microstreaming." While **cavitation effects** at the tip of an ultrasonic scaler can be discerned, they **do not** occur within the root canal. Therefore, **microstreaming** is probably the only effect that is endodontically effective. This involves the continuous elicitation of constant fluid circulation in one direction immediately adjacent to a small vibrating object. Numerous vortices occur, the most rapid at the tip of the root canal instrument. This vortex-elicited effect creates a targeted fluid stream. Acoustic microstreaming destroys bacteria and enzymes.

Studies using models have demonstrated that the **rinsing solution** during the use of ultrasonics only penetrates to the entire length of the root canal if the file vibrates freely. On the other hand, the rinsing solution does not penetrate beyond the first sonic node if interferences with the canal wall inhibit the file vibration. These facts clearly show that the root canal must first be instrumented using the crown-down technique and Gates-Glidden drills or files with a large conicity, so that the ultrasonic file can vibrate freely. Rinsing with ultrasonics during root canal instrumentation is not of significant benefit, but a final rinsing elicits sufficient efficacy of the activated NaOCl solution.

Only K files of size 15 are recommended, and must be prebent to adapt to the canal course, in order to prevent straightening of the canal with ledge formation.

With the use of ultrasonics, freedom from bacteria was achieved during the first appointment in 70% of teeth with apical periodontitis. Simply rinsing with NaOCl led to 50% of the canals being bacteria-free, and rinsing with NaCl led to only 20% freedom from bacteria.

If NaOCl rinsing is supported by ultrasonics, the tissue-dissolving effect in dilacerated root canals is increased. This is even more important because after the first appointment dilacerated canals are never free of tissue debris in all segments, regardless of the instrumentation technique. In addition to debris, segments of the smear layer are also dissolved with ultrasonics. In some cases, even noninstrumented segments of the canal can be freed of accumulated debris using this method; high magnification histology even revealed predentin structures.

Ultrasonically supported rinsing of the root canal is only indicated in those teeth that can be treated at a single appointment, because an interim dressing with calcium hydroxide raises the antibacterial and tissue-dissolving efficacy by over 90% after only one week.

Case Presentation

A Painless premolar exhibits periapical radiolucency; it was treated in one appointment.

B Five percent NaOCl solution dissolves tissue, has antibacterial effects, and therefore is supportive of the mechanical instrumentation.

C The ultrasonic wave consists of nodes with minimal amplitude and balloon-like areas of maximum amplitude; the tip of the file vibrates freely with the greatest amplitude.

D Final ultrasonic rinsing with NaOCl creates a bacteria-free situation in 70% of cases.

E–G Radiographic view at three months, one year, and two years.

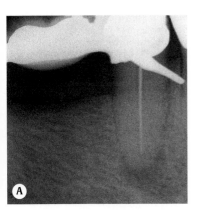

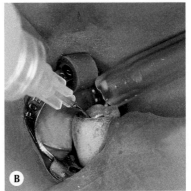

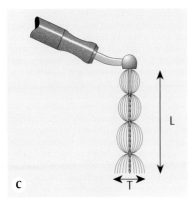

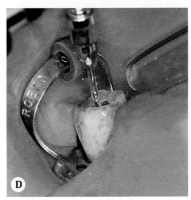

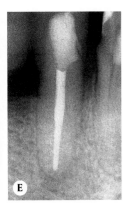

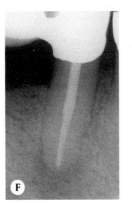

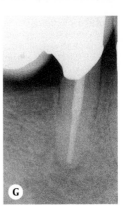

An interim dressing is recommended for infected and necrotic root canals in order to eliminate any bacteria that remain following canal instrumentation, to release or eliminate any endotoxin-elicited inflammation of the periapical tissues, to dissolve any tissue debris in the root canal, as well as to prevent new bacterial colonization (leakage) from the coronal aspect.

Bacteria that survive root canal instrumentation and rinsing proliferate dramatically and quickly between the first and second treatment appointments if the canal remains unfilled. Controlled **asepsis** and effective **root canal disinfection** are essential for successful healing of periapical lesions. Within an infected root canal, there can be as many as 10^8 bacteria per milliliter of canal content, most of them difficult to identify anaerobic microorganisms. Just the mechanical instrumentation of a root canal reduces the bacterial number by a factor of 1000; NaOCl rinses by another 50%.

Medicinal interim dressings play an important role in battling remaining microorganisms that persist following careful instrumentation and rinsing, and to prevent any reinfection.

Even today, the antibacterial properties of **interim dressing medicaments** remain the subject of controversial discussions. Use of such dressings is only justified if the antibacterial activity is significantly greater than the associated cytotoxicity. In order to be effective, the medicament must come into direct contact with the bacteria. Liquid substances are placed into the canal using a paper point, or paste-type dressings by means of a lentulo spiral. Because bacteria will also be present in dentinal tubuli, the interim dressing must have direct contact with the canal wall.

In a study of infected root canals, interim medicament-containing dressings were removed from the canals after one, three, seven, and up to 45 days, and the antibacterial effectiveness was determined. Liquid-dressing medicaments exhibited no antibacterial effect after only one day.

Phenol preparations such as cresol, thymol, and chlorphenol were long touted with regard to microbial reduction and even some degree of pain reduction. However, a benefit/risk comparison revealed only a short-term bacteria-reducing effect in contrast to a long-term cytotoxic characteristic. Formaldehyde and its derivatives exhibit a mutagenic, carcinogenic effect, and can be disseminated throughout the entire organism. With glutaraldehyde, identical adverse effects can be expected. Following contact with tissue fluids, phenol preparations become totally ineffective within a very short period.

If teeth are symptom-free, there is **no indication** for cortisone/antibiotic interim dressings. Cortisone preparations can influence the body's own defense mechanisms negatively, and may also be associated with undesirable systemic side effects. In one clinical study involving corticosteroids applied into the root canal, there was reduction of postoperative pain in teeth with vital pulps, but there was no effect in teeth with necrotic pulps. A comparison among the medicinal dressings formocresol, ledermix, and pure calcium hydroxide showed no differences in the flare-up rate. Mixing calcium hydroxide and corticoids significantly reduces the antimicrobial effects against *Streptococcus sanguis* and *S. aureus*.

An antibacterial interim dressing for infected root canals should only be used as part of a comprehensive antiseptic treatment program. Without mechanical instrumentation as well as copious rinsing of the canal, sufficient asepsis cannot be achieved, even with an antibacterial interim medicinal dressing. Calcium hydroxide is recommended as the interim dressing of choice; however, it cannot eliminate all bacteria.

Case Presentation

A Radiographically obvious apical periodontitis.

B–E Following instrumentation and rinsing with 5% NaOCl and 2% citric acid, Calxyl is applied using paper points, and condensed.

F Appearance three months following canal instrumentation; note the obvious reduction in size of the periapical lesion.

G–I Follow-up radiographs after three, eight, and 18 months.

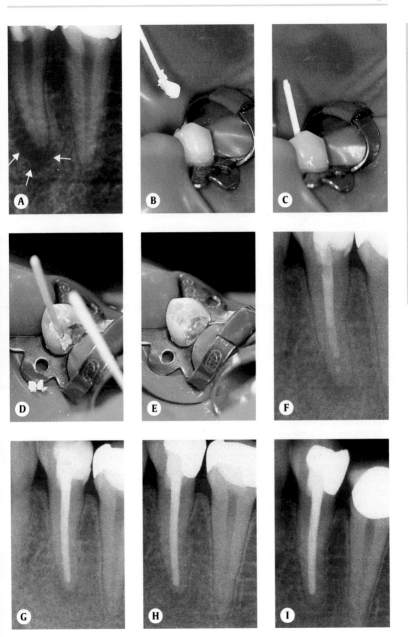

Calcium hydroxide was introduced into dentistry in 1920 (Herrmann). It is a starkly alkaline substance with a pH value of 12.5. In an aqueous solution, $Ca(OH)_2$ dissociates into calcium and hydroxyl ions. The latter possess various biological properties including antimicrobial and tissue dissolving efficacies, inhibition of root resorption and induction of reparative hard tissue mechanisms. Most of the endodontically relevant pathogens (except *E. faecalis*) cannot survive in a strongly alkaline milieu. With direct contact they are eliminated in a short period. In a study by Sundquist, 66% of root canals treated with an application of a phenol-containing interim dressing were free of bacteria; following a calcium hydroxide dressing, 97% of the canals were bacteria-free.

The **antimicrobial effects** of calcium hydroxide result from the release of hydroxyl ions in an aqueous environment; these ions are highly oxidative radicals that react with numerous organic substances. The reaction is nonspecific and intensive, so that the radicals only seldom diffuse away from the point of application, because they have already been quickly bound. The lethal effects result from destruction of the cell membrane, the denaturation of structural proteins and enzymes, as well as DNA damage.

The microbial cell membranes play an important role for the survival of the cell. Hydroxyl ions induce the lipoxidation and destruction of phospholipids, the main componet of the cell membrane. Free fatty acid radicals react with oxygen to form lipid-peroxide radicals that initiate an autocatalytic chain reaction and extensive membrane damage.

In addition, the antimicrobial effect of calcium hydroxide can also occur indirectly. An interim dressing that fills the entire canal can serve as an effective barrier against diffusion, which will inhibit the proliferation of any remaining bacteria and also prevent reinfection from microorganisms in the oral cavity. Temporary fillings with calcium hydroxide can kill remaining microorganisms by means of inhibiting the ingress of nutritive substrates and physically limiting any space for microbial colonization and growth.

The selection of a carrier substance or the solvent for calcium hydroxide powder has particular significance vis-à-vis any antimicrobial and periapical regenerative effects. A mixture with the phenol preparation CMCP, and with glycerin, leads to improved efficacy. The toxic effect of CMCP in such a mixture was interestingly quite low. Other vehicles, in addition to water, include propylene glycol, which is associated with long-term release of OH- and Ca^{2+} ions, as well as control of any pH change.

By itself, calcium hydroxide powder is difficult to introduce into severely dilacerated root canals, and therefore must be mixed with a liquid vehicle. However, if a dilute paste of calcium hydroxide dissolved in synthetic **glycerin** is rotated into a dilacerated root canal by means of a lentulo spiral, the filling is more complete and more homogeneous in comparison to $Ca(OH)_2$ mixtures with sterile water. Using this glycerin paste, the apical third of 50% of canals were tightly closed, in comparison to the aqueous mixture with which **no** canals were filled. For root canals that have been instrumented to file size 25 as well as for severely dilacerated canals, the flexible McSpadden compactors as well as lentulo spiral burs are recommended; using these instruments, the interim dressing reached the apical segment of the root canal in 87% of cases. The Calasept injection technique led to precise placement of the interim dressing in only 48% of root canals, and only 22% were satisfactory after use of the left-turning K files.

Case Presentation

A–C Insertion of calcium hydroxide in a creamy mixture consistency for four weeks. Lentulo spirals were used.

D–F The NiTi McSpadden compactor instruments also effectively insert calcium hydroxide into the root canal. The radiograph one year following treatment clearly reveals complete remission of the periapical radiolucency.

G Commercially available syringes containing calcium hydroxide.

H Calcium hydroxide preparations, some also radiopaque, and the Calxyl suspension that can be diluted.

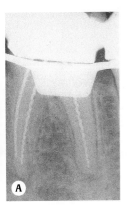

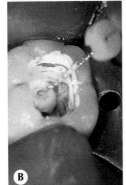

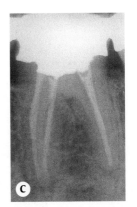

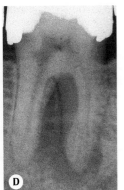

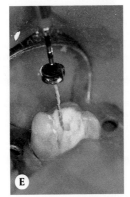

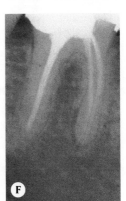

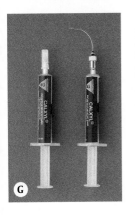

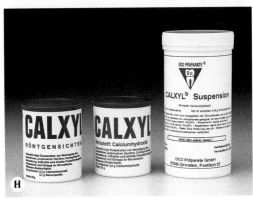

Ionophoresis was introduced into dentistry at the beginning of the 20th century and was the topic of heated and controversial discussion during the 1940s and 1950s. Most recently, **depotphoresis** using copper-calcium hydroxide has been extensively propagated.

In the medical arena, the technique of transporting "loaded" particles within the human organisms with the aid of electric current has been acknowledged for many years. Within the dental specialties, ionophoresis has been proposed for the treatment of osteoradionecrosis, tooth neck hypersensitivity, labial herpes, aphthous stomatitis, anesthesia of skin and mucosa, facial pain syndromes, TMJ problems, and trismus etc.

In 1888, McGrath attempted to disinfect the endodontic system via introduction of galvanic currents. About 80 years ago, the method involving hydroxyl ionophoresis was reinvigorated, and in the 1950s professional journals were filled with creative debates about the possibility of true sterilization of the root canal system.

The concept of **depotphoresis** presupposes complex and interrelated electrical, physical, and chemical processes within the root canal. From a **copper-calcium hydroxide depot** within the root canal, an electric field emanating from a needle electrode has been said to force hydroxyl and copper complexes quickly apically. An alkaline pH value and elevated temperature should dissolve vital as well as necrotic pulp tissue debris (alkaline proteolysis). According to the manufacturer's own statements, these proteolytic products are also forced apically as sterile material and "assimilated" by the body. After exiting through the foraminal delta, the hydroxycuprate ions remain and react to form copper hydroxide, which remains in the apical openings: "The entire canal system is swept clean." Long-acting copper hydroxide remains firmly in the canal system and prevents any reinfection. It is emphasized steadfastly that "in the sense of holistic medicine, no foreign-body elements are employed in the depotphoresis procedure."

A search of the literature, however, reveals no scientific proof for this hypothesis. This is true especially for claims of long-term sealing and sterility.

Profound anesthesia is recommended specifically before employing the procedure, because it permits much more effective current intensities, up to 2.5 mA. However, beyond 5 mA etching or pain can be expected. The manufacturer's own reports include about 10% severe pain, and under certain circumstances even the formation of infiltration or abscess formation! This again speaks against the aforementioned claims of complete assimilation of the bacteria and their toxins.

Following conventional root canal treatment, postoperative complications can be expected in about 5% of patients. Any demonstration of lower statistics cannot yet be attributed to depotphoresis.

In a clinical study by Arnold et al. (1998) of over 2519 root canal treatments, conventional instrumentation led to a success rate of 91.6%, against 8.4% failures. For depotphoresis cases, the success rate was 89.8%, with 10.2% failures. The authors concluded that depotphoresis does not represent a procedure for the optimization of endodontic therapy.

Case Presentation

A The two maxillary central incisors were pain-free, but exhibited fistulae with necrotic pulp tissue.

B Conventional instrumentation was performed, including rinsing with 5% NaOCl solution.

C–E Following determination of the working length, coronal instrumentation was performed, plus a length correction, as well as apical instrumentation to size 30.

F–H Following three months of calcium hydroxide dressings, the root canals were filled; the intraoral fistulae had closed, and the radiolucencies had begun to disappear.

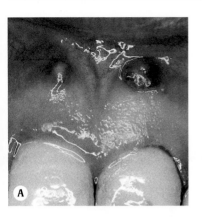

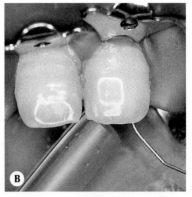

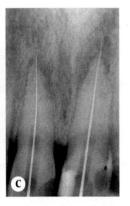

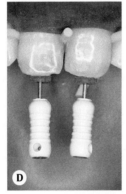

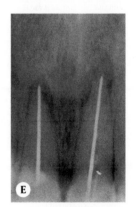

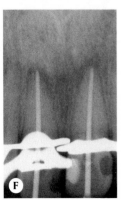

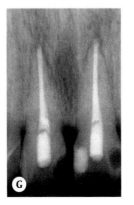

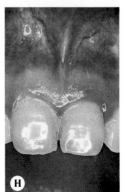

There is a direct correlation between the expanse of the periapical lesion, the number of **bacterial strains**, and the number individual bacteria within the root canal; teeth exhibiting large periapical lesions are associated with more different types of bacteria as well as higher bacterial density.

The periapical lesion results from a **nonspecific infection**. Microbiologic experiments have demonstrated that various bacteria are capable of eliciting periapical lesions in various ways. Experiments have also shown that combinations of bacteria, or specific bacteria, play a role in the development of periapical abscess; among these are the black-pigmenting, gram-negative anaerobic bacteria.

How can these bacteria be eliminated most effectively? The answer is clear: by means of mechanical instrumentation (cleansing), supported by antibacterial solutions (rinsing), as well as the use of antibacterial interim dressings.

One of the most *incorrect* premises regarding treatment of acute apical periodontitis is that the tooth should be **left open** between two appointments following **trepanation**, regardless of the amount of purulent material that was released. There are many facts that speak against leaving a canal open: The canal is contaminated additionally, food debris will be impacted into the canal, and otherwise avoidable appointments for treatment of the tooth must be planned. The length of time during which the tooth is left open and the number of attempts to render the tooth symptom-free are correlated positively with each other.

The goal of every successful endodontic treatment is to eliminate the bacteria and their metabolic by-products that are responsible for the existence of a periapical lesion, and to create a condition that prohibits reinfection. This is accomplished by mechanical instrumentation (cleansing), antibacterial rinsing, and an effective but biocompatible interim dressing for the time between the treatment appointments.

In cases of acute apical periodontitis, pus should be released **via the root canal**.

This will be successful in most cases, but in exceptional circumstances, e.g., with a blocked canal or with reduced host-response capacity, an **incision** through the oral soft tissues may be required. If the decision is made to leave the canal/tooth open, the working length must be determined and the canal must be completely instrumented. The patient must rinse often with saline solution in order to prevent any blockage of the trepanation opening. At the most, 48 hours later, the patient must be reappointed for closure of the coronal opening.

If **drainage via the root canal** is possible, following trepanation the coronal pulp is removed, the access is expansively enlarged, copiously rinsed with NaOCl and instrumented into the apical segment using a size 15 Hedström file.

If no pus flow occurs, instrumentation 1 mm beyond the apex can be performed. After additional canal rinsing, the tooth is left open for ca. 20 minutes, instrumented up to file size 25, and then finally rinsed with citric acid. Using a lentulo spiral, calcium hydroxide is inserted, the tooth is closed, and the patient is reappointed five days later for complete instrumentation. At this time, instrumentation is performed up to the apical constriction to file size 30 (or larger), and closure with well-condensed calcium hydroxide suspension (which can remain in the canal for four to 12 weeks). If the patient remains symptom-free, the canal can be definitively filled at the third appointment.

If the intraoral soft tissue swelling is small, this treatment is usually sufficient; if the swelling in the region of the tooth is large and fluctuant, an additional soft tissue **incision** is recommended. There is usually no necessity for systemic antibiotic coverage.

Case Presentation

A/B Extraoral and intraoral swelling in the maxillary anterior segment; the patient reported radiating pain.

C Following trepanation and careful coronal expansion, there was copious pus release after deeper preparation of the root canal.

D After rinsing with NaOCl and finally with citric acid, Calxyl was inserted as an interim dressing.

E Initial situation revealing the periapical lesions.

F Radiographic view three months following Calxyl application.

G Radiograph taken 1.5 years later reveals no apical radiolucency.

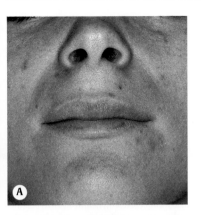

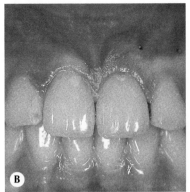

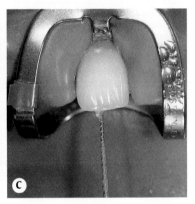

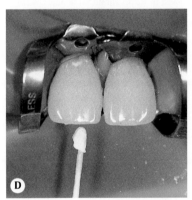

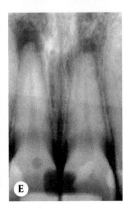

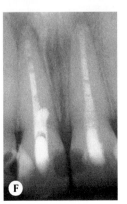

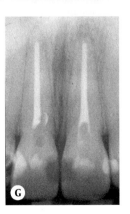

Because dilacerated root canals will not be completely freed of tissue debris by chemo-mechanical instrumentation, the interim dressing is even more important. The anaerobic conditions within a closed root canal do not inhibit the tissue-dissolving properties. Even after seven days, calcium hydroxide exhibits a very good **tissue dissolution effect**, which in contrast to the initially rapid dissolving by sodium hypochlorite, continues more slowly and continuously.

Pulpal soft tissue will dissolve within three hours in 0.5% NaOCl if the solution is changed every 30 minutes. In Ca(OH)$_2$ suspension, the tissue is completely dissolved after 12 days. If the tissue is pretreated for seven days in Ca(OH)$_2$ pulpal tissue will be completely dissolved in NaOCl within 60 minutes. A single one-week calcium hydroxide dressing dissolves any noninstrumented odontoblastic layer; a four-week dressing erodes even the predentin layer.

Light microscopic examinations have demonstrated that a one-week interim dressing and subsequent rinsing during instrumentation with NaOCl cleans the isthmus of mesial mandibular root canals completely; the additional use of ultrasonics does not improve the cleansing efficacy.

Hydroxyl ions diffuse through dentin with a pH maximum, if the interim dressing is *in situ* for at least three weeks. After only 24 hours, a maximum of pH 10.8 was achieved on the internal dentinal canal wall. The longer the interim dressing is allowed to work in the root canal, the more favorable is the regeneration within the inflamed periapical tissues. In a controlled histologic study of the short-term and long-term effects of calcium hydroxide on experimentally induced apical periodontitis, after one week of treatment osseous regeneration was observed in only 50% of patients. If the medicament was changed weekly for a 12-week period, *every* case exhibited complete regeneration with cementum apposition.

When calcium hydroxide is used as an interim dressing, even large periapical lesions exhibit complete **regeneration** in 82% of patients three years later; in 18%, radiographs reveal only minor reduction or even persistence of the apical periodontitis. The greatest reduction of periapical lesions occurs within the first year. Initial signs of regeneration can be detected in the radiograph at the earliest after 12 weeks; in digital films, as early as three to six weeks.

The occurrence of **pain** is much more frequent with small periapical lesions as opposed to larger lesions. The prophylactic administration of antibiotics did not reduce pain following endodontic treatment, when compared with a placebo.

There are some reports that the **dentin matrix** and some tissue components may neutralize the antimicrobial properties of calcium hydroxide. In a comparative study of the reduction of antibacterial effect of three medicaments, calcium hydroxide was inactivated when employed with dentin, hydroxylapatite, or bovine serum albumin. In addition, in the presence of dentin powder, calcium hydroxide exhibited no effects against *Enterococcus faecalis.* Only the final rinsing with an **EDTA** solution or with **citric acid** inactivated the dentin matrix and led to a satisfactory antibacterial action against these test microorganisms.

Case Presentation

A   Clinical photo of a fistulous canal into which a gutta percha point had been inserted.

B   The radiograph reveals a large periapical radiolucency.

C   Instrumentation of the root canals to the apices.

D   Following NaOCl rinsing, instrumentation and final rinsing with citric acid, calcium hydroxide was placed and condensed into the canal.

E   Only three weeks following instrumentation of the root canals, the fistula closed spontaneously.

F   Radiograph three months later.

G/H Radiographs taken one and two years later exhibit significant periapical regeneration.

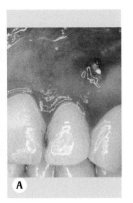

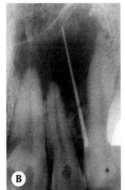

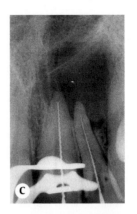

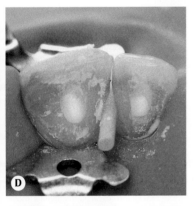

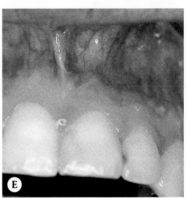

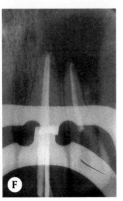

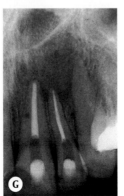

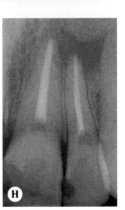

In teeth exhibiting periapical lesions, one must differentiate between:
- a primary infection with necrotic pulpal tissue
- a secondary infection following endodontic treatment failure.

In cases of an **endodontic primary infection**, the microflora consists primarily of obligate anaerobic microorganisms. In such cases, **calcium hydroxide** is indicated as the intermediate dressing in order to eliminate all relevant bacteria.

The microflora in cases of **endodontic failure** are quite different from those of a primary infection; facultative anaerobic microorganisms predominate. In a study of 54 endodontic failures, retreatment of the root canal procedure was performed. A microbiologic evaluation revealed significantly fewer bacterial species in endodontic failures, when compared with primary infections. In more than one-third of all cases, only a single species could be detected. On average, there were 1.7 species types per root canal. Gram-positive species also dominated in cases of persisting periapical lesions. *Enterococcus faecalis* was the most prominent microbe in endodontic failures; this is a bacterium that is very difficult to eliminate using conventional methods.

In cases of endodontic failure, **mechanical instrumentation** combined with **NaOCl** will not lead to total absence of bacteria. Even the use of calcium hydroxide as an interim dressing does not exert sufficient antibacterial effect against *E. faecalis* in the root canal.

Several authors declare that the use of calcium hydroxide as an interim dressing prepares the basis for the continuing viability of this individual microorganism, because all other endodontic-specific microbiota are killed. In contrast to other microbial species, enterococci can persist viably as a single species within the root canal.

Calcium hydroxide has been shown to be most efficient when it is mixed with **chlorhexidine** or **camphor-paramonochlorphenol** (CMCP) instead of with physiologic saline or sterile water. When used for five minutes as a rinsing solution, both 0.2% chlorhexidine, as well as 5% NaOCl, are equally effective antibacterially against *E. faecalis*. With a seven-day treatment, however, chlorhexidine gel was clearly superior when used as the single medicament. When root canals were rinsed with chlorhexidine immediately before filling, they were free of bacteria 35 days later, while canals rinsed with NaOCl exhibited bacteria after only 24 hours.

Most scientific studies have demonstrated no difference between the antimicrobial efficacy of 0.2% or 2% chlorhexidine solutions, but a 2% solution appears to eliminate microorganisms more quickly. Indeed, with a one-hour working time, even a fungicidal effect was observed.

Chlorhexidine may be superior to sodium hypochlorite, but it exhibits no tissue-dissolving effects; chlorhexidine should be employed during retreatment of endodontic failures, in addition to NaOCl. In such cases, one may mix the interim dressings with chlorhexidine, but some controversy exists as to whether there will be any elevation of antibacterial effect. One study demonstrated that a **mixture of calcium hydroxide and chlorhexidine** exhibited a pH value of 12.0, identical to that of aqueous calcium hydroxide.

The best antibacterial effect against *E. faecalis* was a **mixture of calcium hydroxide with glycerin and CMCP**.

Caution: Before placing an interim calcium hydroxide dressing (**not** before placing the definitive root canal filling!), the dentin matrix should be inactivated by rinsing with citric acid.

Case Presentation

A The radiograph reveals a mandibular molar containing a broken instrument and an insufficient root canal filling; note the periapical lesion.

B The fractured instrument was removed with the help of ultrasonics.

C Following dissolution of the remaining gutta perch using eucalyptol, the patency of the canal was checked.

D The canals were rinsed with 5% NaOCl and 0.2% chlorhexidine solution.

E/F The Ca(OH)$_2$-CHX dressing was removed using an H file.

G/H Three months later the canals were definitively filled. Apical regeneration is clearly visible.

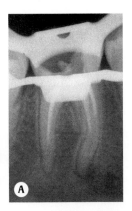

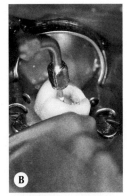

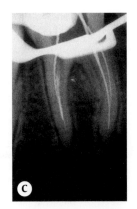

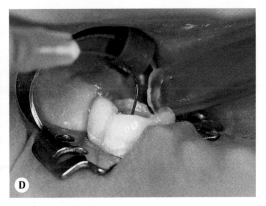

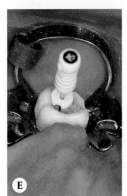

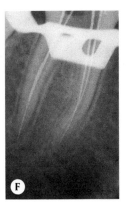

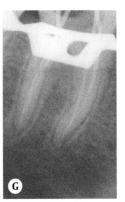

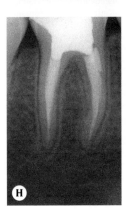

In view of the beneficial effects of calcium hydroxide in the root canal, gutta percha points **containing** calcium hydroxide represent a new innovation. These points contain about 50% calcium hydroxide, 40–45% gutta percha as well as 4–10% barium sulfate, titanium dioxide, waxes, and oils. The points are indicated for the **temporary medicinal treatment** of the canal.

In an aqueous milieu, these points appear to release hydroxyl ions, so that within a few minutes the pH increases. In isotonic saline solution, it achieves pH 11. The problem with invitro measurements, however, is that few definitive conclusions regarding the actual clinical situation can be drawn. On the one hand, substances used within the canal can have contact with tissue fluids that are physiologically buffered, and on the other hand, dentin itself exhibits a not insignificant buffering capacity. The release of hydroxyl ions in Tris-HCl buffer was therefore not surprisingly very low. In contrast to dissolved potassium hydroxide powder, there was no significant elevation of the pH value.

In double-distilled water, the alkalinization was also smaller than with other calcium hydroxide-containing substances. With gutta percha points, after two hours a maximum pH of 9.5 was measured, which fell to 8.1 after 24 hours. The comparative value for Rheogan was always 12.0. In addition, in other solvents such as artificial saliva and bovine serum, the pH increase was slight (up to ca. 8.5).

Measurements of the **alkalinization** of root canal dentin demonstrated that placement of calcium hydroxide-containing gutta percha points led to no or minimal increase of the pH in dentin. Compared with controls, a significant elevation of pH was measurable only immediately adjacent to the root canal dentin after 24 hours, and was no longer detectable after three days. The gutta percha points release so few hydroxyl ions in the root canal that these are neutralized by the **buffering capacity** of the dentin matrix.

Even in comparisons of canals with an intact smear layer and canals whose smear layer had been removed, there was no significant difference with regard to pH elevation after several days.

Thus, within the root canal, and assuming similar buffering systems, only liquid calcium hydroxide suspensions can elicit a pH increase and therefore exhibit significant antibacterial effects. It was demonstrated that not all of the calcium hydroxide present in the gutta percha points was released, only that portion on the surface. Nevertheless, the consistency of the points changes significantly, and the material adheres to the internal canal wall; after extended periods, it is difficult to remove from the canal.

One promising technique is use in combination with an aqueous calcium hydroxide suspension. The suspension can be rotated into the canal using a lentulo spiral or the McSpadden compactor, with subsequent insertion of a calcium hydroxide-containing gutta percha point that is pushed laterally, and somewhat apically, and then compacted. This ensures good contact with the dentin surface, and the calcium hydroxide can better exert its antibacterial effects.

Case Presentation

A Mandibular first molar with acute pulpitis and a periapical radiolucency. Following trepanation, pus exuded from the opened canals.

B The canals were instrumented using the crown-down technique, and then rinsed with 5% NaOCl and with citric acid solution.

C During drying of the canals, no additional pus was visible on the paper points; a calcium hydroxide suspension was rotated into the canals.

D/E The suspension is pressed against the canal walls by insertion of the calcium hydroxide-containing gutta percha point.

F Definitive root canal filling, three months later.

G Two years later, complete remission of the periapical radiolucency is apparent.

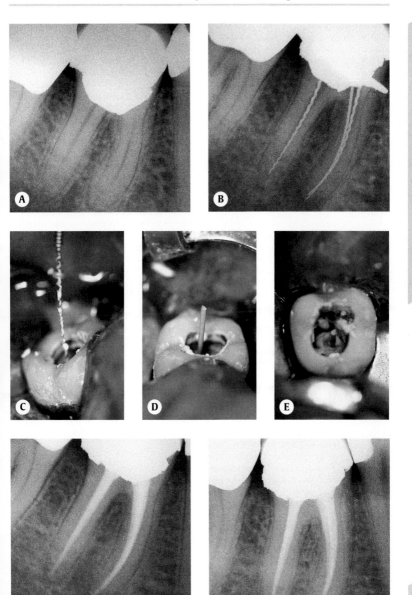

It is still not known even today how much time is required for a calcium hydroxide dressing to sufficiently disinfect the root canal. Clinical studies with cultures extracted from root canals have provided varying results: Following a three-month calcium hydroxide dressing, 90% of canals examined were free of bacteria; in a second study, 97% of the canals were bacteria-free after only a four-week interim dressing. In contrast, in 26% of examined patients, there was still a persisting infection demonstrated after 2-week dressing applications. Two additional studies showed a 92.5–100% bacterial elimination after only a one-week application, and a third reported bacteria in only 22.6% of canals after one week.

All of the studies cited above demonstrate that **calcium hydroxide** certainly reduces the number of bacteria in infected root canals, but that it is not always able to eliminate all microorganisms completely. A very likely explanation is the sometimes quite variable **total** antibacterial treatment. This involves:

- type and duration of the mechanical cleansing (instrumentation)
- type, amount and concentration of the rinsing solutions employed
- the solvent or vehicle used to mix the calcium hydroxide powder.

A recent study showed that the best antibacterial efficacy of calcium hydroxide is achieved when it is mixed with **CHKM** (a phenol) and **glycerin**.

Even in cases in which bacteriologic samples from the canal resulted in no cultures, endodontic failure can still occur. This can occur when bacteria remain in isthmuses, dentinal tubuli, or ramifications that were not reached by the interim dressing material. In addition, it has been demonstrated experimentally many times that calcium hydroxide is ineffective against *Enterococcus faecalis*. This species can survive even in highly alkaline environments, apparently via a mechanism that pumps protons intracellularly, therefore maintaining the cellular cytoplasm in the acidic range. In an actual clinical study by Peters and Wesselink (2002), no improved results occurred after the use of calcium hydroxide dressings following root canal treatment of asymptomatic teeth with necrotic pulps and periapical radiolucency. In a total of 39 treatments, 81% exhibited complete remission of the periapical radiolucency 4.5 years following treatment of the root canal in one appointment and without interim dressings. In contrast, in canals treated for four weeks with a calcium hydroxide interim dressing, only 71% were successful. Interestingly, the success rate was 87.5% even in canals with a positive bacteriologic test result.

It is critical to note that, in these clinical studies, there was **no** additional rinsing with **EDTA or citric acid solutions**.

If the canal is rinsed with one of these solutions before placing the dressing, the treatment success rate will be clearly better in the one-appointment treatment group. These results emanated from a controlled histologic animal experiment, and demonstrated more favorable results with longer interim dressing treatments (Holland et al. 2003).

In summary, calcium hydroxide consistently reduced the number of microorganisms, but was only successful if the dentin matrix was inactivated before application.

In **symptom-free teeth**, a one-appointment treatment is almost always the most reasonable approach.

Case Presentation

A Teeth 46/47 were associated with intermittent symptoms of pulpitis, but no periapical pathology was observed.

B Blood emanating from the canals indicates an essentially vital pulp without infection.

C–E Instrumentation and filling of the root canals of tooth 47 at one appointment.

F/G At a second appointment, tooth 46 was instrumented and immediately filled. Both teeth were subsequently symptom-free.

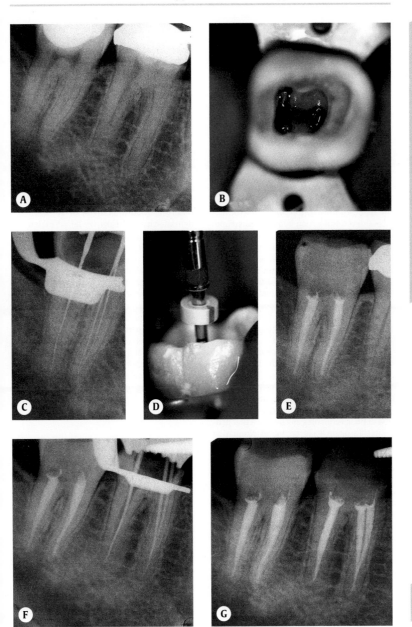

The temporary closure must tightly seal the **coronal trepanation opening** between appointments, in order to prohibit any bacterial penetration into the root canal system. Two of the most frequently used materials are Cavit and IRM cement:

- In one study of sealing effectiveness, Cavit allowed penetration through the filling material to a depth of up to 4.3 mm and marginal penetration of 4.4 mm.
- Using IRM, a dye substance penetrated only 0.5 mm marginally but along a length of 4.9 mm.

Based on these results, a temporary restoration thickness of 3.5 mm is inadequate. Even the application of a cotton pellet upon the medicinal interim dressing beneath the temporary filling must be avoided. A **thickness of over 4 mm** is the goal; this can only be achieved by direct application onto the root canal orifices. Identically severe saliva penetration occurred three months after root canal fillings with a ca. 3 mm thick IRM restoration as with teeth that were left open coronally. Such restorations must be replaced after one month *in situ* because sealing failure increases with time.

With IRM cement, evidence of discoloration of a cotton pellet placed directly beneath a 5 mm thick filling at the floor of the cavity was observed twice as often compared with Cavit. If the canal orifices are directly sealed by the temporary filling material, contamination of the interim dressing by saliva that penetrates through leaky crown or restoration margins is less likely to occur.

The type of temporary filling material can negatively influence the seal of the definitive restoration. IRM cement, Cavit, Dycal, but also Grossman cement lowers the bonding strength of a composite material to dentin by one-half of the control value.

On the other hand, the type of temporary dressing within the root canal does not significantly influence the sealing properties of the restorative materials. Neither eugenol nor formocresol nor chlorphenol elicit any higher penetration through or beyond the restoration.

It has long been known that **recontamination** of an already treated root canal almost always occurs from the coronal aspect, and that a poorly sealing restoration (or secondary caries) can lead over time to failure despite optimum root canal instrumentation and filling. In a study of saliva contamination, canals were instrumented *in vitro* and filled, but not closed coronally. A group of control teeth was sealed coronally with wax. Following the set reaction of the sealers, the apices of the teeth were placed into nutritive substrate solution and the access cavities were filled with human saliva. In the teeth that were filled with gutta percha and without any coronal closure, bacterial growth at the apex was observed after only 48 hours. In the control group, not a single case of bacteria penetrating apically was observed. Following lateral or vertical condensation using a sealer, the length of time for complete penetration was maximally 48 days.

If the tooth was not closed coronally, after a maximum of three months less than half of the teeth still exhibited an impervious filling. Over the long term, best results were achieved with adhesive composite resins, followed by glass ionomer cement. With only a one-month interim dressing, two-thirds remained coronally impermeable, i.e., no penetration could be observed along the restoration margin. As a result of these studies, the temporary dressing should not be left in place longer than **four weeks**, also because of possible coronal leakage of the temporary restoration.

Case Presentation

A/B Following instrumentation, rinsing and drying, calcium hydroxide is condensed.

C/D Coronal closure was accomplished using a more than 4 mm thick layer of glass ionomer cement. After four weeks, the filling is removed and the temporary dressing is checked.

E/F Initial and measurement radiographs.

G Six months later, the periapical lesion is significantly reduced in size.

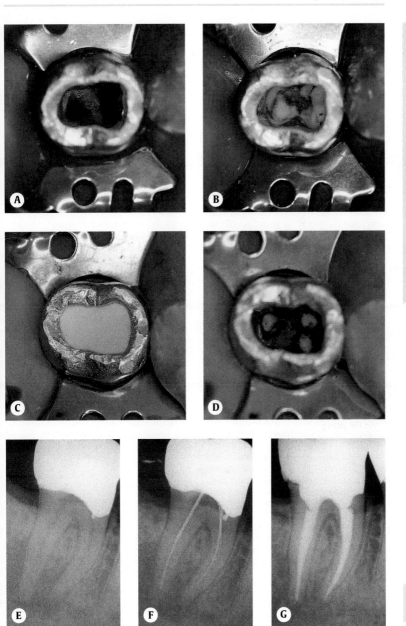

The final procedure of endodontic therapy is the creation of a hermetic filling of the root canal using material that is non-irritating to tissue.

Thorough and complete mechanical instrumentation and shaping of the root canal are the most important prerequisites for endodontic success. The root canal filling should render the tooth as inert as possible vis-à-vis the entire organism; it should also prevent any reinfection, or any proliferation of microorganisms that might have been left within the canal.

If **resorbable pastes** are forced beyond the apical foramen, the result can be acute inflammation, resorption of adjacent alveolar bone, and in rare cases even abscess formation. If the canal is filled with **resin cement** (**polyketone base**) the periapical tissue exhibits inflammation with predominance of macrophages and foreign body giant cells; in rare cases, an *acute* inflammatory reaction may also be observed. If the canal is overfilled with this material, necrosis as well as cementum and bone resorption of varying expanse will occur. After 80 days, a connective tissue capsule forms around the extruded material; cementum resorption seldom occurs, but a pronounced foreign body reaction is often observed.

Root canal fillings employing the **formaldehyde-containing cement N2** elicit a foreign body reaction, and within adjacent tissues areas of necrosis and accumulation of leukocytes are observed. This filling material undergoes resorption, and is therefore distributed via the periapical soft tissues throughout the body.

An **ideal root canal filling material** should not irritate the periapical tissues, should tightly close the root canal laterally and vertically, and should maintain a constant volume, i.e., not shrink within the root canal; in addition, the material must not enhance or otherwise favor bacterial growth, should be bacteriostatic as far as possible, while maintaining biological compatibility and nontoxicity; the material should be easily and rapidly sterilizable, must not discolor the tooth, and should be radiopaque. In addition, a **root canal sealer** should not set too quickly, should bind well to both dentin and the master point after the set reaction, should be insoluble in tissue fluid,

and should only minimally expand upon setting. These "ideal" properties cannot be achieved in a single formulation, and therefore compromises have been made with most root canal filling materials, as well as with filling techniques.

Root canal filling with **gutta percha points** and a sealer is the most reliable method for long-term biologic compatibility. Well-accepted and time-proven **methods of application** include:
- lateral condensation
- vertical condensation
- thermomechanical condensation.

Gutta percha points consist of:
- 19–45% gutta percha
- 33–61% zinc oxide
- 1–4.1% wax
- 1.5–3.1% heavy metal salts.

Most gutta percha points are of the **beta form**, which are distinguished from the alpha form by a **predetermined melting point**. This is dependent upon the composition. Alpha gutta percha begins to soften beyond 65–79°C, and then starts to flow without any chemical decompensation. These properties are taken advantage of by the Obtura system. Upon cooling, shrinkage is ca. 2–2.6%, which can be compensated by manual follow-up condensation (cf. vertical condensation).

The root canal can be definitively obturated if the tooth is pain-free, not percussion sensitive, not adjacent to soft tissue swellings, free of obvious fistulae, and the instrumented canal is dry and odor-free.

Illustrations

A ISO-normed and color-coded gutta percha.

B Gutta percha points from various manufacturers.

C Non-normed gutta percha and finger spreaders for lateral condensation.

D Hand spreaders with increasing sizes.

E Finger pluggers with flat ends.

F Hand pluggers with 5 mm graduations for use in vertical condensation.

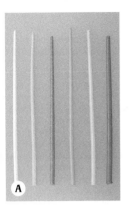

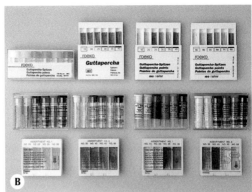

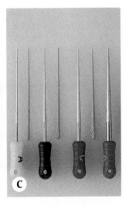

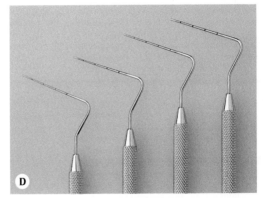

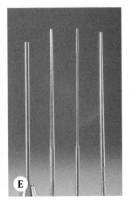

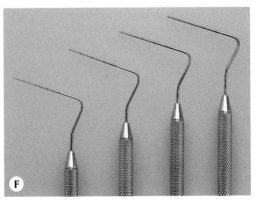

Following complete mechanical instrumentation of the root canal, a final rinsing is performed, but the canal is not yet completely dried; this simplifies test insertion of the spreader and the gutta percha master point. An appropriate **finger spreader** is selected, which should make contact with the canal wall 1mm short of the working length. The length can be marked with a rubber stop. In accordance with the size of the apical master file, the gutta percha master point is selected, and its length and position in the root canal are carefully evaluated radiographically.

The length of the **gutta percha point** is registered by means of an indentation using a small forceps. Then the gutta percha point is coated with the **sealer** (AH-plus, 2-Seal) and slowly inserted into the root canal to the coronal reference point. Then the nitinol spreader is inserted with sufficient pressure up to the indicated stop, left in place for at least 15 seconds, and then removed with a slight rotatory movement.

If the spreader will not penetrate deeply enough into the canal, this is usually due to the course of the root canal. It may also be due to an improper choice of spreader size. If the condensation instrument sticks in the middle third of the canal, Gates-Glidden drills should be used coronally for additional expansion, or a smaller spreader can be selected. Wedge-shaped spreaders are not indicated because of the danger of a vertical tooth fracture.

During condensation using the spreader, two things occur: **lateral deformation** (compression), and also a further **apical positioning** of the gutta percha. However, the elongation is minimal (average 0.29mm), and at the tip of the gutta percha point the displacement averages only 0.69mm.

Into the space created by the lateral condensation of the master point, size 20 accessory gutta percha points are inserted. The tip of each additional gutta percha point is dipped into the sealer before insertion into the canal. The same finger spreader is inserted into the canal between the gutta percha point and the dentin canal wall, then pressed apically as possible to the measured depth, and then removed using rotatory movements; in this way the accessory gutta percha is condensed onto the canal wall and onto the master point.

Then a third gutta percha point is laterally condensed using the spreader, pressing it against and into the first points. The finger spreader is used for condensation until it can only penetrate to the coronal third of the canal and until the root canal filling is homogeneous. Before the gutta percha is severed coronally, a radiograph is taken with the spreader *in situ* to check the position and depth. This permits any necessary corrections.

In order to prevent discoloration of the tooth crown by components of the root canal filling material, a heated instrument must be used to sever the filling material 2mm apical to the cementoenamel junction. A plugger marked appropriately for the desired length can be useful for final condensation. After removing any excess gutta percha, the coronal 4mm of material remains soft and can be further condensed into the canal entrance. After placing a coronal restoration, the root canal filling is checked with a final radiograph.

Illustrations

A The spreader is inserted adjacent to the master point to 1mm short of the apical foramen.

B/C Insertion and subsequent lateral condensation of the gutta percha master point.

D Because of the irregularity of the canal walls, the gutta percha master point does not completely fill it.

E Following initial condensation, the gutta percha point is deformed and pressed against the canal walls.

F A sealer-coated secondary gutta percha point is inserted into the cavity.

G The schematic depicts the laterally condensed gutta percha point and the spreader.

H The cross-section schematic shows the third accessory gutta percha point (pink) following lateral condensation.

I Condensation of the individual gutta percha points leads to a homogeneous mass, whose percentage composition of sealer is less than 5%.

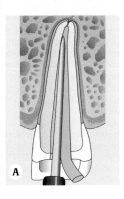

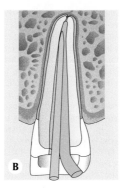

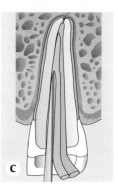

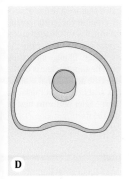

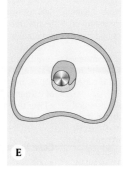

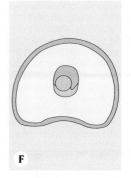

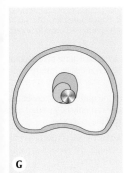

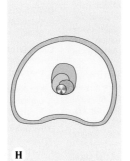

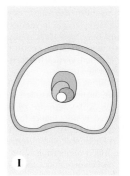

The actual filling of the root canal begins with the selection of the gutta percha master point. Gutta percha must not be overmanipulated because otherwise it will become fragile and brittle, no longer permitting sufficient condensation. This is the result of light-accelerated and heat-accelerated changes in the crystal lattice structure. Gutta percha that has not undergone dessication is much easier to condense. **Softer** gutta percha is easier to condense.

Before adapting the **gutta percha master point**, the appropriate spreader is selected. The sealing capacity of any root canal filling depends upon the shape and depth of penetration of the **spreader**. The distance between the tip of the gutta percha point and the D11-spreader with its conical, wedge-shape is more than 2 mm within the root canal. On the other hand, an ISO-standardized finger spreader can reach up to 1 mm from the tip of the gutta percha point. This results in a more homogeneous root canal filling.

Once the master point has been accurately measured radiographically, it is again removed from the canal, and the canal is rinsed and dried.

In about one-half of cases, the lentulo spiral adequately applies the sealer. However, if the gutta percha master point is coated directly with the sealer and then slowly inserted into the canal, optimum sealing can be achieved.

In mildly dilacerated root canals, **nickel-titanium finger spreaders** generally effect better sealing than hand spreaders. The danger of a vertical tooth fracture during condensation is relatively low, but is dependent upon the spreader design. In comparison to standardized finger spreaders, conical spreaders cause 4× more frequent dentin deformation with expansion. **Vertical fractures** occurred in 5% of obturated teeth.

During condensation in dilacerated root canals, the nitinol spreaders appear to be advantageous because in comparison to steel spreaders they induce lower loading forcers. In straight canals, on the other hand, no difference was observed in terms of canal sealing and force application.

Following initial condensation of the gutta percha master point, additional points are condensed onto the canal wall. If the root canals are obturated using ISO-normed accessory gutta percha points of size 20, using finger spreaders, the filling will be significantly more homogeneous, and overfilling, or crease creation, will not occur. Nonstandardized fine accessory gutta percha points are associated with overfilling in 30% of cases, and the fillings very frequently exhibit folds, cavities and nonhomogeneous areas.

During lateral condensation, a sealer is absolutely necessary; without this, effective closure of the canal is significantly poorer. The biological acceptability of the root canal filling is determined, in most part, by how much sealer actually comes into contact with the periapical tissues. The goal is a relationship of about 95% biologically inert gutta percha to 5% resorbable sealer.

One study revealed that with use of Proco-Seal as sealer and dipping the gutta percha points into chloroform, lateral condensation resulted in 94.5% gutta percha 1 mm from the root tip. However, after filling, increasing shrinkage occurred. The film thickness of the sealer also influences the actual canal sealing. AH-26 and Sealapex seal better at a thickness of 0.3 mm, while Kerr-Sealer performs best at a layer thickness of 0.05 mm.

Case Presentation

A–C Following radiographic evaluation of the master point, the point is coated with sealer and inserted into the canal with up and down movements.

D With a size 30 finger spreader, the gutta percha points are condensed onto/into each other.

E The tip of each additional gutta percha point is dipped into sealer and then inserted into the canal.

F Condensation of the gutta percha continues until the spreader can only be inserted into the middle third of the root canal.

G Following removal of the excess gutta percha using a heated spatula, the remaining material is vertically condensed.

H/I Visual (clinical) and final radiographic check of the complete root canal filling.

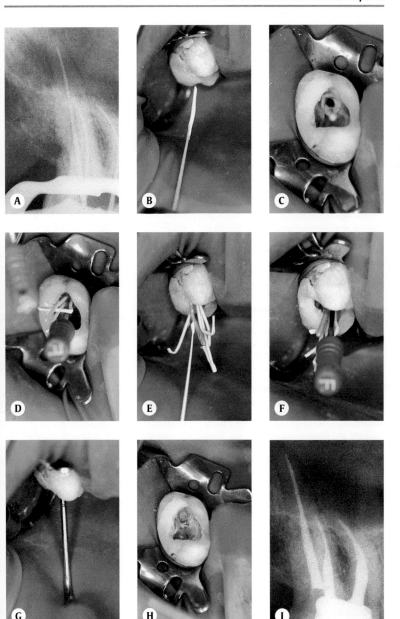

The most common **causes** for undesired **extrusion** of gutta percha beyond the root apex include:

- excessive instrumentation beyond the apical constriction
- unexpected resorptive defects
- iatrogenically elicited defects such as perforation, notching or apical funnel creation
- excessive force application during condensation
- the use of a gutta percha master point that is too small.

To avoid these potential problems, a radiograph of the master point *in situ* is essential. During the extended process of condensation, another radiograph should be taken. Resorbable root canal filling cements are irritating to vital tissues; only gutta percha is biologically inert. Nevertheless, a sealer is necessary because gutta percha by itself cannot hermetically seal the root canal, and it does not adhere to the canal walls. If small amounts of gutta percha and sealer extrude from the apex, the tissue reaction is usually mild. A circumscribed inflammatory reaction will surround extruded sealer particles; around the gutta percha point a thin connective tissue capsule with fibroblasts and some lymphocytes will form.

In cases of **overinstrumentation** with widening of the apical constriction, the try-in of the gutta percha master point becomes of critical importance. An advantage of the lateral condensation technique is that some corrections are still possible even during the filling procedure. Nevertheless, the danger of extrusion of excess sealer paste into the periapical tissues is relatively high when using the lentulo spiral.

If the **master point** is too long, it can be shortened by several millimeters using a scalpel on a sterile glass slab; this effectively increases the diameter of the tip. The new tip is smoothed and rounded by light rolling. The gutta percha point is then **dipped into a softening solution** and adapted to the individual root canal shape and form. The apical 5 mm of the gutta percha point is either dipped for five seconds into chloroform, 15 seconds into halothane, or 25 seconds in eucalyptol. After only one second, gutta percha absorbs 0.35 mg

of solution, but 62% of it evaporates after three minutes. Nevertheless, 20% of the chloroform remains on the surface of the point. During try-in of the master point, the canal must not be completely dry, because otherwise the gutta percha point will stick to the canal wall. The point is inserted into the canal up to the length marking, and then removed about 15 seconds later. After drying the canal, the sealer-coated gutta percha point is condensed, resulting in a well-adapted root canal filling.

If the gutta percha master point cannot be inserted to the **full working length**, the cause is usually canal blockage by an accumulation of dentin chips in the apical third of the root canal. Such canal blockage can be removed using RC Prep and Hedström file #20 with rotatory movements. Chelators are also indicated to overcome canal obliteration and blockage. Rinsing the root canal with citric acid or with a chelator enhances the penetration of the sealer into dentinal tubuli. **Injected** gutta percha flows more readily into the tubuli following removal of the smear layer. Interestingly, sealer will penetrate adjacent dentinal tubuli up to 300μm, even if the smear layer is intact. The smear layer does not inhibit penetration of sealer into the tubuli.

Any accumulation of dentin chips is the result of improper rotation of the K file, and/or improper rinsing with NaOCl solution. Once the dentin chips are loosened with the small Hedström file and chelators, and then copiously rinsed, the apical master file must again be employed to the full working length for complete instrumentation. Using the small H file, the canal is once more instrumented, and the gutta percha master point can then be assessed radiographically.

Case Presentation

A–C If the master point is too long, a larger one is dipped into eucalyptol and again tried.

D–F It is also possible to shorten the measured point by 2 mm and then soften it before insertion. During the condensation procedure, an additional radiograph can be taken to check the position.

G–I If the point is too short, the canal must be rinsed with EDTA and reinstrumented.

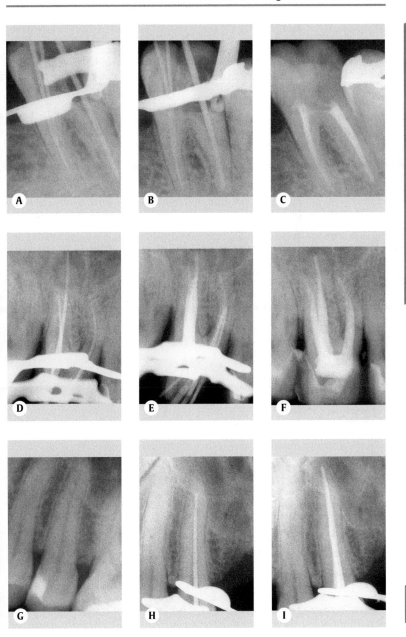

The original form of Thermafil was developed by Johnson (1978) and introduced onto the market by Tulsa USA. The licensed product was DensFil (Dentsply-Caulk), and after further development, Thermafil (Maillefer) and Soft-Core (Loser) were marketed.

The new **Thermafil-plus points** are size-matched to the new nickel-titanium files, and are available in conicities from 4–10% (new in the NiTi-GT system). The coating of the gutta percha is a plastic substance that exhibits a small notch; this simplifies subsequent removal for preparation of a build-up restoration ("post and core").

Using the Thermafil system, root canals can be filled with gutta percha quickly and with reduced effort. The system consists of standardized plastic points that are coated with **alpha gutta percha**. The gutta percha softens upon warming, and the root canal can be filled in a single procedure. However, following instrumentation to size 25, there is a relatively high occurrence of underfilling the canal. With instrumentation to size 35, the point almost always reaches the apex, but some cases of overfilling may occur. In the study by Clark and El-Deeb, the frequency of overfilling was greater with the Thermafil system than with conventional lateral condensation.

During insertion, some gutta percha may be partially scraped away so that the plastic carrier point comes into direct contact with the periapical tissues. Care must be taken in the clinical routine to avoid insufficient insertion depth in narrow or dilacerated root canals, or in some cases massive overfilling.

In contrast to conventional lateral or vertical gutta percha condensation, with the Thermafil technique no master point radiograph is taken. For accurate length determination, a "measurement point" (verifier) is inserted into the canal to the established working depth, and the definitive Thermafil point is selected in the same size, but is not actually tried-in.

It is recommended that the smear layer be eliminated by rinsing with EDTA or citric acid before filling the root canal, so that the softened gutta percha can flow without inhibition into the microretentions. After thoroughly drying the root canal, a paper point is used to apply a small amount of sealer (AH-plus, 2-Seal) onto the coronal root canal walls. If sealer is applied to the canal walls using a lentulo spiral, the danger of extrusion at the apex during insertion of the Thermafil point is very high.

The Thermafil point is placed into the **warming oven**, where the gutta percha of appropriate size is heated. Thereafter, the Thermafil point is slowly inserted into the root canal continuously in one motion without rotation. Closure and impervious sealing at the apex are directly related to the precision with which the coronal expansion during instrumentation of the root canal was performed. Finally, a special high-speed bur (Thermo-Cut) is used to remove the excess gutta percha that extends coronally out of the root canal.

If, subsequently, the tooth is to be prepared for a post-and-core, the canal orifices can be widened using the high-speed "Post-space bur," and any Thermafil debris can be rinsed from this area.

Case Presentation

A Instrumentation of the straight root canal is performed up to the apex to size 35.

B Checking the working length in a radiograph.

C Application of a small amount of sealer into the coronal third of the root canal.

D Application of sealer.

E The heated Thermafil point is slowly inserted into the root canal.

F Using a Thermo-Cut bur, any material emanating from the canal coronally is excised.

G Special oven for heating the gutta percha-coated Thermafil point.

H After heating, the Thermafil carrier is removed from the oven and inserted into the root canal up to the rubber stop.

I The Thermafil point is severed and removed at the level of the canal orifice. The radiograph depicts a somewhat short but homogeneous root canal filling.

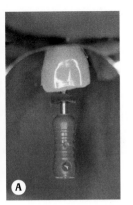

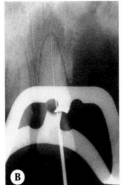

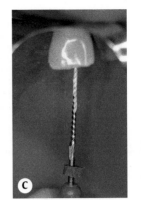

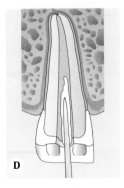

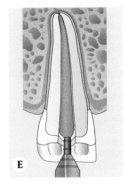

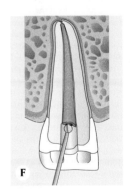

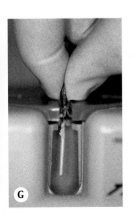

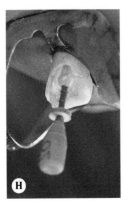

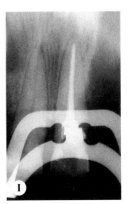

The instrumentarium consists of a nine-piece **plugger set**. The instruments of sizes 8–12 begin with a diameter of 0.4 mm, and the diameter increases by 0.1 mm per instrument. The pluggers are graduated at 5 mm intervals. This permits checking the length, even when the instrument is within the root canal. Three pluggers are used that are slightly smaller than the diameter of the root canal at corresponding depths.

The smallest plugger should extend to 4–5 mm coronal to the **apical foramen**. In the coronal third, the broadest plugger must function without touching the canal walls; a narrower plugger is used for the middle third of the canal. The pluggers are selected before try-in of the master point. A **spreader** heated in an alcohol flame may be employed to warm the gutta percha. A better method, however, is the use of a heating device, for example the Touch 'n' Heat 5004 (Analytic Technology), which warms the gutta percha to a maximum of 45°C and progressively softens the points.

Following canal instrumentation, a non-standardized **gutta percha point** of size "medium" is selected, which corresponds to the shape of the conically prepared root canal and which fits the canal due to its corresponding conicity. The master point is tried-in to the full working length and the position is checked with a radiograph. Then the point is removed from the root canal, and should exhibit some apical resistance during removal ("**tug back**"). Before the gutta percha point is finally and definitively inserted, the tip is trimmed by 0.5 mm.

For vertical condensation, **Kerr Sealer** is recommended; it hardens within 15–30 minutes and, in comparison to other sealers, provides the thinnest film thickness as well as a very good flow capacity and viscosity. Once the sealer has been applied and the master point inserted, one initiates the **down-pack** phase with the hot removal of gutta percha at the level of the canal orifice and initial condensation using the largest plugger. Then the Touch 'n' Heat probe is inserted into the gutta percha, the heating element is turned off at the handpiece, and after a short moment the probe is pulled out of the gutta percha. The smaller plugger can then be used more deeply in the root canal to condense the heated gutta percha, which is distributed three-dimensionally 4–5 mm deeper, and also into any lateral canals.

During the final heating procedure, the heated probe reaches the apical area. The thinnest plugger is used to maximally 5 mm short of the apical constriction, serving to fill any fine branchings of the apical delta during condensation. The plugger is used with firm, apically directed force until the gutta percha has cooled; this prevents any shrinkage during the cooling phase. The danger of extrusion is relatively low if the master point has been shortened by 0.5 mm and precisely adapted to the root canal.

After conclusion of the first phase of vertical condensation (down pack), the next phase is either the adaptation of a post build-up, or the root canal can be completely filled coronally with gutta percha (**back pack**). For this purpose the gutta percha "pistol" Obtura II is used; this heats the gutta percha to 160°C. The plasticized gutta percha leaves the injection cannula at a temperature of 47°C to a maximum 81°C, without causing injury to the adjacent marginal periodontal tissues.

Illustrations

A Selecting the three plugger sizes.

B Measuring the nonstandardized master point.

C Heated severing of the coronal gutta percha.

D Initial vertical condensation (down pack).

E Renewed warming of the gutta percha point.

F Condensation of the gutta percha with a small plugger in deeper regions of the canal.

G Following conclusion of the "down pack," the coronal segment is filled using the gutta percha pistol.

H Subsequently the gutta percha is condensed via vertical condensation.

I Final root canal filling.

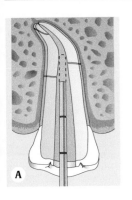

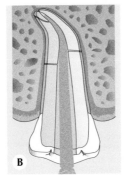

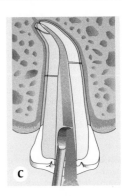

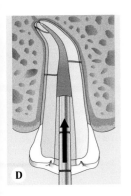

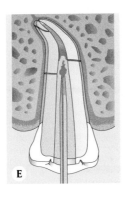

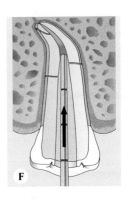

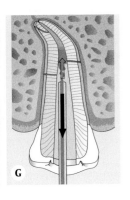

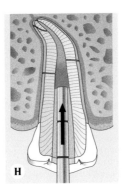

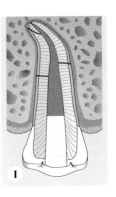

The root canal contains **ramifications** and **lateral canals** that communicate in the furcation region or apically with the periodontal tissues. Every outlet from the root canal is a possible site of penetration by bacterial metabolic products from a necrotic pulp. The tendency for regeneration of periapical lesions of endodontic origin is dependent upon a myriad of parameters. One of these is the complete "**filling technique in three-dimensions**," which was developed by Schilder.

Heating makes possible a three-dimensional root canal filling with bioinert gutta percha. The gutta percha conducts heat 4–5 mm. Over this distance, condensation can be performed.

Repeated heating of the gutta percha point to 40–45°C causes softening over the entire length of the point, even apically. This renders the gutta percha condensable. During the cooling phase from 45–37°C, vertical condensation is performed. This both adapts and stabilizes the gutta percha in all three dimensions.

Although anatomic peculiarities such as multiple canals and ramifications correlate with the number of endodontic failures, the main causes for failure are incomplete instrumentation, poor shaping, and incomplete obturation of the primary canal. One clinical study demonstrated that, in cases exhibiting large periapical lesions, the long-term bone regeneration success after vertical condensation of biologically inert gutta percha was 97.9%.

Case Presentation

A Try-in of the thinnest plugger; it should be inserted up to the apical dilaceration of the canal without scraping the canal walls. The distance to the apical constriction should be maximally 4–5 mm. A medium-sized plugger should passively reach the middle third of the canal. The length is marked with a rubber stop, or one can note the length marking on the surface of the plugger. The plugger selection ensures that, during the condensation procedure, the instrument compacts only the plasticized gutta percha and does not bind on the canal walls. Otherwise, additional vertical condensation is not possible.

B An additional radiograph can be used to check the expected depth of penetration of the narrowest plugger.

C The master point is shortened apically by 0.5 mm, coated with sealer, and inserted into the root canal. Using a heated excavator, the excess gutta percha is trimmed away, and the coronal-most 4 mm of gutta percha are warmed using a heated probe (Touch 'n' Heat device). When the spreader is removed, it carries with it a small amount of gutta percha and this makes possible even further apical condensation.

D Dipping the broad spreader in cement powder prevents it sticking to the softened gutta percha. Short, circumferential strokes upon the heated gutta percha effect the condensation. Finally, the plugger is forced in the apical direction, and one senses the consolidation of the gutta percha filling. Pressure applied by the plugger, as well as apical counterforce of the nonheated gutta percha, also forces the plastic filling material into lateral canals.

E This combination of heating and vertical condensation of the gutta percha is repeated three or four times until the thinnest plugger can be inserted 4–5 mm from the previously determined working depth. There is little danger of extruding gutta percha beyond the apex if the root canal has been instrumented conically, the master point has been well adapted, the temperature does not exceed 45°C, and the heated probe does not insert beyond 4 mm short of the apical foramen. Following the initial phase of vertical condensation (down pack), a radiograph is taken to check the filled segment of the root canal.

F The cannula of the gutta percha pistol makes contact with the apical gutta percha filling, and expands the surface. Upon careful withdrawal of the cannula, a small amount of gutta percha is deposited. The medium-sized plugger compresses the gutta percha apically, and then condensation is performed circumferentially in order to achieve a homogeneous root canal filling.

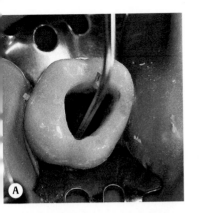

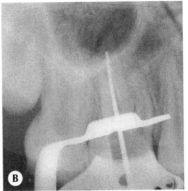

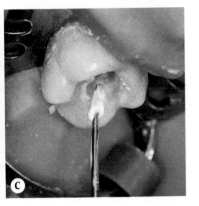

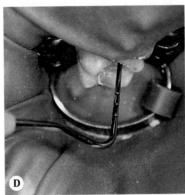

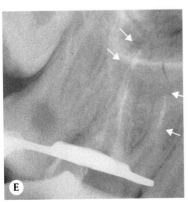

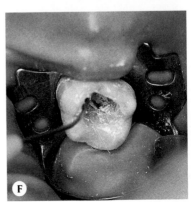

Within a single endodontic practice, 116 endodontically treated teeth had to be extracted within an 11-year period. Of these teeth 59.4% teeth were extracted for prosthetic reasons, and this is a clear indication that endodontic therapy is not complete until prosthetic reconstruction is successful. In addition 46.5% of the failures were crown fractures, and in 8.6% root fractures occurred due to improper placement of post build-ups. In addition, 32% of the teeth were extracted for periodontal reasons; in only 10% was the **endodontic therapy** responsible for the failure.

Frequency and quality of root canal fillings were studied by Klimek et al. (1995) using radiographs from 500 patients during 1991. The homogeneity of the fillings was satisfactory in only 50% of cases. Over 45% of the teeth exhibited a periapical radiolucency.

It is imperative to differentiate between **retreatment** of an inadequate root canal filling in a tooth that is **free of clinical symptoms** or radiographic alterations, vis-à-vis teeth exhibiting clinical and/or radiographic **symptoms**. The indications for retreatment include clinical symptoms such as fistula formation, swelling, pain, percussion sensitivity, and discomfort during mastication, as well as apical lesions that become larger or do not **decrease** in size. Retreatment following an inadequate endodontic procedure should be targeted toward eliminating infection and preventing any reinfection.

The primary etiology of endodontic failure is bacteria remaining within the root canal system. In one histologic study, six out of nine root tip biopsies exhibited microorganisms in nontreated apical segments of the root canal; four contained several bacterial species. In other cases, without evidence of bacteria, a giant cell granuloma was apparent, as evidence of a foreign body reaction to the filling material.

In cases of endodontic **failure**, the microbiologic profile within the root canal is often different from that before initial therapy. In a study by Pinheiro et al. (2003), 51 out of 60 examined teeth exhibited bacteria. In 28 root canals, only one individual bacterial species was present; in eight canals, two species, and 15 teeth exhibited a polymicrobial colonization of three or more bacteria species. Interestingly 57% of the organisms were facultative anaerobes, and 83% were gram-positive. Most frequently observed were *Enterococcus, Streptococcus,* and *Actinomyces*. **Enterococcus faecalis** was the most common microorganism (53%). If an endodontic failure is retreated, and if this bacterium (*Enterococcus faecalis*) was present in the canal, the success rate is 66%; the success rate for retreatment of canals without this microorganism is 75%.

The clinical success for retreatment is significantly less than that for initial endodontic treatment, which can exceed 90%.

According to Grossman, the **reasons for retreatment** include incorrect diagnosis, poor prognosis, technical difficulties, and negligent initial treatment. In the Washington study, 76% of the failures were related to **clinician error**, e.g., incompletely instrumented or incompletely filled canals, perforations and severe overfilling, as well as fractured instruments. In 22%, the etiology was traced to improper case selection.

The primary **indication for retreatment** is an endodontically treated tooth with periapical radiolucency that has not regressed within four years or which has appeared since initial endodontic treatment. If further prosthodontic procedures are planned, inadequate root canal fillings must be retreated even if there are no clinical or radiographic symptoms.

Case Presentation

A/B The molar exhibits poor prosthetic treatment (overhanging crown margins, secondary caries) and apparent partial filling of the coronal pulp chamber.

C/D The caries was removed, the crown margins were properly adapted, and the root canals were reinstrumented and then rinsed with NaOCl and Chlorhexamed.

E/F Following an interim dressing with calcium hydroxide-CHKM-glycerin, the canal was obturated. The radiograph exhibits healthy conditions three years later.

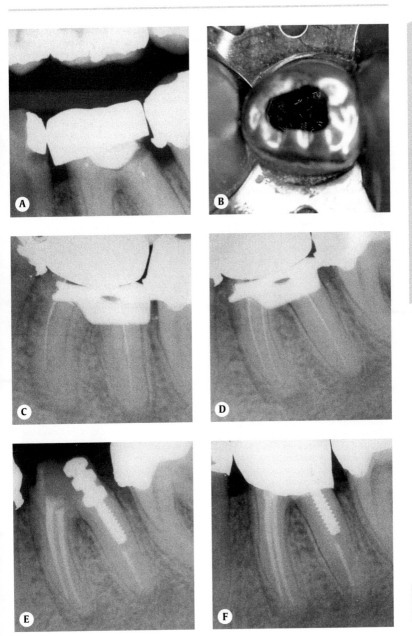

Fractures of endodontically treated teeth are often blamed on reduced physical characteristics of dentin. In fact, however, the dentin of endodontically treated teeth does not exhibit physical characteristics or resistance properties that differ in any way from the dentin within vital, healthy teeth. Nevertheless, the shape and expanse of the **access cavity** as well as the subsequent coronal restoration may influence or enhance the danger of fracture. Following an MO (mesio-occlusal) preparation, the load-bearing capacity of dentin was reduced to 81% of normal, and following MOD preparation, only 61%. The creation of an endodontic access cavity reduces overall coronal rigidity by one-half.

The dentin of endodontically treated teeth is in no way more susceptible to fracture than the dentin within vital teeth. Neither the dehydration of dentin nor the age of the patient has any significant influence upon the degree of dentin deformability. The removal of the pulp chamber roof and the marginal ridge(s) nevertheless considerably reduces the resistance capacity. Molars fracture only after loading of 341 kg, but an MOD preparation reduces molar resistance to 222 kg. Teeth with endodontic access cavities and MOD preparations will fracture with only a 121 kg loading.

The altered **mechanical properties** of a prepared tooth elevate its susceptibility to fracture. Over an observation period of 20 years, the restoration of endodontically treated teeth with amalgam generally led to less than satisfactory results. Teeth with an MOD restoration exhibit fractures more frequently than teeth with intact marginal ridges. At the end of the period of observation, only 30% of maxillary and 40% of mandibular premolars remained intact. Not surprisingly, teeth with DO or MO restorations were associated with a significantly better survival rate (80%).

While a perfect MOD restoration with amalgam may reduce the danger of fracture by increasing the rigidity from 61 to 82%, a **cast partial crown** "capping the cusps" increases this value to 125%. Capping the cusps increases the rigidity of mesial cusps by 175%, but distal cusps only by 102%. These facts lead to the conclusion that endodontically treated posterior teeth must be restored with at minimum a cast partial crown capping the cusps in order to guarantee long-term protection against tooth fracture.

An **inadequate coronal restoration** can play a critically important role in the occurrence of **endodontic failure**. With a perfect coronal restoration and excellent endodontic treatment, treatment success can be expected in 91% of cases; however, the long-term success rate with an imperfect coronal restoration sinks to only 44%, even with acceptable endodontic treatment.

Incompletely sealed areas of crown margins can permit penetration of saliva and **bacteria**, and then to the development of renewed necrosis within the root canal system. Invitro studies of cases of inadequate temporary or even definitive restorations revealed severe reinfection of the root canal system after only seven days. In another study, **all** endodontically treated root canals became contaminated by saliva and bacteria within 30 days.

Particularly noteworthy is that **temporary** restoration with zinc oxide-eugenol cement was associated with an elevated occurrence of coronal leakage, in comparison to **definitive** restoration. The danger of coronal leakage increases with increasing time between root canal filling temporary closure, and the subsequent definitive restoration of an endodontically treated tooth.

Case Presentation

A The molar exhibits a fistula. Six years previously, the crown was temporarily seated. Since then, the patient did not appear for definitive seating of the crown.

B The radiograph reveals large periapical lesions that extend into the area of the bifurcation.

C Mechanical root canal instrumentation, followed by rinsing with 5% NaOCl as well as 0.2% chlorhexidine solution.

D Note the obvious remission of the osseous lesion following three-month treatment with calcium hydroxide-CHKM dressing.

E Closure of the fistula after only three weeks.

F Clinical view one year following completion of treatment and definitive seating of the crown.

G/H One-year and two-year check-up radiographs exhibiting further remission of the periapical lesions.

I Four years later, a small periapical radiolucency persists on the distal root tip.

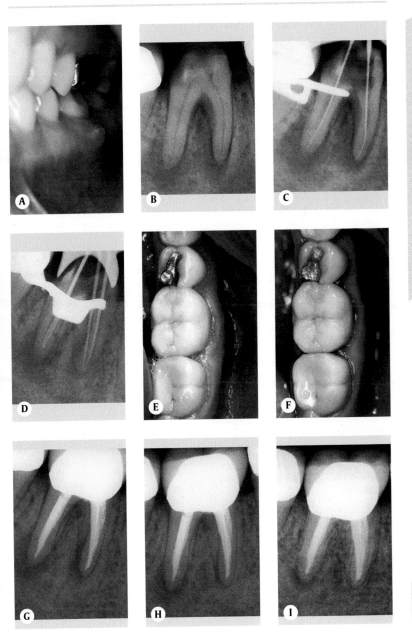

If the tooth has been restored with a crown and a post build-up (custom cast "post and core" or prefabricated post), these must be removed before any attempt at endodontic retreatment. Removal of the crown permits better observation of the tooth anatomy and preparation of a more favorable access cavity. In the absence of a restoration, evaluation of diagnostic radiographs with regard to perforation in the furcation region, length of a silver point filling or obliteration in the region of the canal orifice is simplified. In addition, vertical fractures and the expanse of carious demineralizations are easier to assess without the crown *in situ.*

Preparation for a post build-up weakens the dental hard tissues. If the post has to be removed, tooth fracture can occur. The removal of a screw-type post is usually less dangerous, but the risk increases proportional to the contact surface.

The use of **ultrasonics** reduces the post's adhesion to the root canal wall surface, thus making removal of the post considerably easier. Before attempting to dislodge the post, remnants of cement must be loosened using a pointed ultrasonic scaler tip. In exceptional cases, diamond-coated or carbide burs may also be used.

Parallel-wall posts cemented with zinc phosphate cement 4 mm within the canal should be exposed to the ultrasonic for up to eight minutes to loosen them, and then removed with a forceps using about 1 kg of force. On the other hand, even **60 minutes** treatment with devices that operate in the **sonic region** cannot even partially loosen such posts, and therefore sonic devices are not indicated. The removal of posts from the root canal required 35% less force following the use of ultrasonics.

After removal of the post, the **canal orifices** must be identified with the help of magnifying loupes or a surgical microscope; subsequently, the root canals are reinstrumented. Simultaneously, an optical control of the cavity floor must be performed to identify any **fracture lines,** which are an indication of a vertical fracture resulting from removal of the post; detection of fracture lines negatively tempers the prognosis for success of the endodontic retreatment. Application of methylene blue stain (Canal Blue) can better reveal any fracture lines.

Overlooked primary canals or unidentified apical ramifications etc. are primary causes for endodontic failure.

About 40% of mandibular incisors have two root canals; but in only 1% are there separate apical foramina.

During retreatment, both orthoradial and excentric radiographic projections must be used in order to better portray any anatomic variations.

An additional root canal will be found in ca. 84% of maxillary first premolars, and in 58% of maxillary second premolars.

In addition, 8% of first premolars will exhibit three or more primary ramifications. Mandibular premolars exhibit the most complex root canal system: 31% of first and 11% of second premolars have two primary ramifications, and 3% have a third primary canal. More than 20% of anterior teeth and 50% of posterior teeth exhibit numerous ramifications. These canal **branchings** are almost impossible to instrument mechanically, but adequate and copious rinsing with sodium hypochlorite can cleanse them effectively. During endodontic retreatment, such ramifications are usually closed with sealer paste or dentin chips, making complete tissue removal virtually impossible.

Case Presentation

A The molar exhibits a full crown restoration, a screw-type post, and root canal fillings that are short of the apices. Pain was the reason for retreatment, even though no radiographic pathology was apparent.

B Following removal of the build-up, all residual cement must be removed.

C Subsequently the post is loosened using a broad ultrasonic tip to a depth of about 2 mm.

D/E Under the surgical microscope, the floor of the cavity did not exhibit any fracture lines, but a fourth canal orifice was detected adjacent to the distal root canal.

F Final radiograph following retreatment. The patient was completely symptom-free.

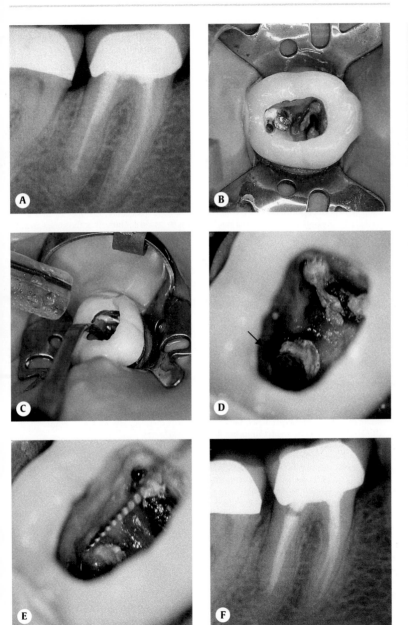

The **success of retreatment** of a canal previously treated with gutta percha depends on the quality of condensation, the length of the filling and the severity of dilaceration of the canal.

Coronal portions of the gutta percha are softened with a heated instrument and removed. Then, Gates-Glidden drills are used to remove 3–5mm of gutta percha from the canal, creating space for the application of a **dissolving solution**. Dissolving the gutta percha is indicated if the filling is well sealed and does not extrude apically. Subsequently the filling material is carefully removed, first using Hedström files and finally nickel-titanium files with a 6% conicity.

The most effective dissolving agent for gutta percha is **chloroform**. However, chloroform has recently been categorized as a possible carcinogen. Maintaining the solution in a syringe reduces the danger for the dentist and his/her assistant to an acceptable level. In the interim, other dissolving agents such as eucalyptol or halothane have become available with equally good dissolving characteristics.

Eucalyptol is less irritating than chloroform. However, if it extrudes beyond the apex, a tissue reaction is elicited. Chloroform will dissolve a gutta percha filling to a depth of 1.1mm; eucalyptol extends only to 0.9mm and **halothane** up to 0.8mm. Within 70 seconds, all three of these dissolving agents permit the penetration of a Hedström file into the softened gutta percha up to a depth of 10mm.

The average **time for retreatment** varies depending upon the sealer used; seven minutes with AH-plus, and more than 10minutes for Ketac-Endo. Gutta percha can be also removed with various motor-driven NiTi instruments; in the coronal third of the canal, Gates-Glidden drills as well as Orifice-Shapers (ProFile system, red or yellow) or also GT files with 6 or 8% conicity. This speeds the clinical procedure and creates space for the dissolving agent, while providing improved access to the apical segment of the root canal. The speed for these instruments is higher, and can reach 500rpm. After applying the dissolving agent, speed is reduced to 300rpm, because the softened gutta percha is less resistant. The instruments must be repeatedly removed from the canal and all gutta percha debris removed using a gauze square soaked in eucalyptol.

When using hand instruments, one must exercise special care to avoid creating ledges within the root canal.

During the removal of gutta percha, the root canal is rinsed exclusively with eucalyptol. Once the region that is 2mm removed from the apical constriction has been achieved, the clinician may begin definitive shaping of the root canal. During this procedure, the canals are rinsed not only with 5% NaOCl solution but also alternatively with 0.2% chlorhexidine, because one must anticipate the presence of *Enterococcus faecalis*.

Following determination of length, the canal is completely instrumented mechanically, and rinsed finally with **citric acid**. With a retreatment procedure, the root canal should not be sealed definitively at the same appointment. Calcium hydroxide mixed with sterile saline solution can be used as a temporary dressing, but even after one week neither *E. faecalis* nor *Fusobacterium nucleatum* will be eliminated from the dentinal tubules, whereas a mixture of calcium hydroxide, CMCP and glycerin effectively kills these bacteria after only one hour.

Case Presentation

A The maxillary premolar was sensitive to biting force.

B The canal orifices are readily visible.

C Using a Gates-Glidden drill, the gutta percha is removed to a depth of about 4mm.

D A small amount of eucalyptol is then injected into the space created.

E The gutta percha is completely removed ...

F ... and the canal length is determined radiographically.

G Following rinsing with NaOCl and CHX, a dressing of calcium hydroxide-CHKM-glycerin is placed.

H Final radiograph three months later; the patient was painfree.

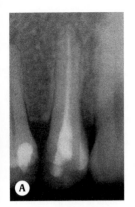

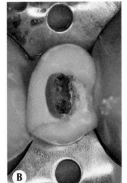

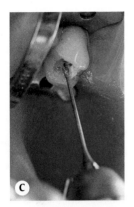

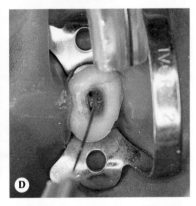

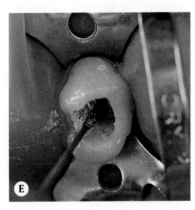

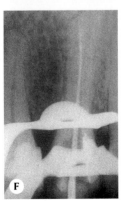

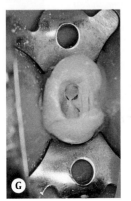

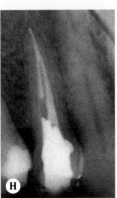

Silver points have been used in endodontics for over 100 years. The underlying premise during the development of silver point root canal fillings was the **antibacterial effect** of silver. Even small amounts of silver or mercury completely kill bacteria *in vitro*. This led to the term "oligodynamic effect" (Greek: **oligos**, little; **dynamos**, force). The assumption was that bacteria release soluble metal salts from the surface of the silver point, and that these have a toxic effect.

As early as 1921, a mixture of silver and copper was utilized as a root canal filling paste; in 1929, a silver point was used in conjunction with a silver-containing paste. However, in 1936, Grossman proclaimed that the results of invitro studies cannot always or completely be related to the clinical situation within a root canal, which raised doubts concerning any true oligodynamic effect within the canal. Grossman favored silver points from a purely practical perspective: They are easy to place, even in narrow and dilacerated canals. Later, numerous experiments confirmed the **oligodynamic effect**, but it has never been clarified whether this effect also occurs under invivo conditions. Following initial reduction of the bacterial load, bacterial proliferation frequently occurred after only a short period.

Comparative studies revealed that root canal fillings with silver points were up to 13× less impermeable in comparison to lateral condensation of gutta percha. Because it is very difficult to instrument the apical region of a dilacerated root canal into a round/oval form, silver points can achieve excellent length control, but a definitively poorer lateral seal.

In the apical region, the silver point must be completely covered by sealer, because otherwise the point will come into contact with tissue fluid and corrosion will occur. This can lead to complete **disintegration** of the silver point. Corrosion products such as silver sulfide, chloride, sulfate and carbonate occur not only on the point itself but also in dentin and within the adjacent periapical soft tissues.

In many cases, such degradative processes lead to clinical failure. Nevertheless, in a study of root canal fillings that had been *in situ* for at least five years, the success rate for gutta percha fillings (85%) was not different from that with silver point fillings (83%). Failure often occurred much later than with gutta percha fillings. The success rate for retreatment is 69% for silver point fillings, similar to that for gutta percha.

When attempting **retreatment of silver point endodontic fillings**, one must exercise care that the coronal section of the point not be severed during trepanation of the coronal segment. Only the use of an **ultrasonic scaler** will loosen the filling material at the depth of the silver point. Frequently it is possible to remove the corroded silver point from the canal using a diamond-coated forceps, even without additional attempts to loosen it. If this is not successful, the point is exposed as deeply as possible. Then a broad ultrasonic scaler is used around the coronal end of the silver point to loosen it.

Case Presentation

A Because the marginal seal was inadequate, Hedström files could be inserted along the silver point into the apical region of the root canal, and using a rotatory motion the point could be grasped and removed.

B It is also possible to use a spoon excavator to loosen the silver point.

C Using the Masseran armamentarium, the coronal end of the silver point is grasped, and then loosened ultrasonically. The point can then be removed.

D A clearly discolored and painful anterior tooth exhibits a silver point filling and condensed gutta percha, without periapical radiolucency, but exhibiting mild lateral resorptions.

E After dissolving the gutta percha, a Hedström file is inserted apically.

F–H Three files were inserted: When rotated 90° to each other, the silver point was loosened.

I Following removal of the silver point, the canal is then reinstrumented, rinsed, and then filled following a four-week period with a temporary dressing in situ.

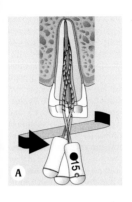

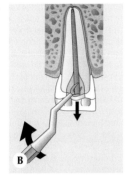

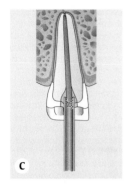

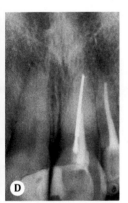

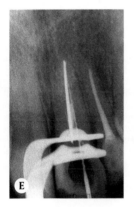

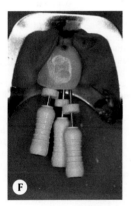

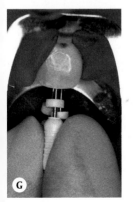

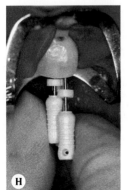

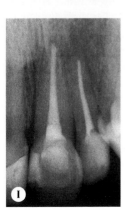

Fracture of a file during canal instrumentation is surely one of the most unpleasant incidents. Radiographic studies have shown that instrument fracture occurs in about 6% of cases. Orthograde retreatment is very difficult in most cases; it is time consuming, and often a hopeless endeavor depending upon how deep within the canal the fracture occurred. There is no single therapy that works in all cases. In-vitro studies using ultrasonics suggested a success rate of 79%; *in vivo*, the broken instrument was successfully removed in 67% of cases.

Before any attempt at retreatment of an endodontic failure, the patient must be thoroughly and completely **informed**. During the removal of an inadequate root canal filling, perforation of the root may occur, or instrument fracture, or extrusion of filling material, or a broken instrument fragment beyond the apex. The patient must consider the possible alternatives, and must decide whether he/she is prepared to participate in an attempt to maintain a tooth, with full understanding of the time commitment and costs, as well as likely mental stress.

Broken instrument fragments should be removed from the root canal whenever possible, and the canal must be reinstrumented.

Anatomic factors will influence the chances for success or failure of attempts to remove broken instruments; additional influencing factors include the type, length and position of the instrument fragment. In addition, the type of fracture, the clinical routine of the dentist, the diameter and cross-sectional shape of the canal, as well as the techniques and instruments that are available, will play important roles. The **success rate** for removal of broken instruments was higher if the case involved maxillary teeth, or if the fragment was lodged in the coronal third of the canal, or if the instrument fractured coronal to any dilaceration of the canal, or if the instrument fragment was longer than 7 mm, and finally if the broken instrument was a reamer or a Lentulo spiral.

Every retreatment attempt must begin with a thorough analysis of the type of fragment and its position and location in the root canal. In the case of instruments that were forced excessively into the canal, the friction against the dentin walls will be high, bringing with it less likelihood of successful retreatment. On the other hand, if the instrument ex-

perienced a stress fracture, friction is low and the chances of removal are good. Fractured spiral drills are sufficiently flexible; they can be surrounded and removed relatively easily.

Using Gates drills sizes #1 and #2, the canal is widened up to the site of the instrument fragment. Then the coronal portion of the root canal must be additionally widened by successive use of Gates drills #3, #4, #5, and eventually also #6 to permit free oscillation of an ultrasonic spreader.

If instrument fracture occurred in the apical third of a narrow and dilacerated canal, or if the instrument cannot be loosened because of a high level of friction, an attempt can be made to circumnavigate the fragment, carefully widen the canal and fill it with gutta percha, leaving the fragment *in situ*.

Fractured stainless steel instruments that are left in the canal are relatively inert and do not exhibit corrosion even after two years. On the other hand, silver point fragments will corrode and therefore **must** be removed.

Following the removal of an insufficient root canal filling, acute reaction can be expected in 13% of cases, even in teeth that were clinically pain-free initially. Therefore, following every retreatment and reinstrumentation, a calcium hydroxide dressing must be placed and left *in situ* for four weeks.

Illustrations

A Note the two broken instrument fragments in the mesial root, apical to the canal's dilaceration.

B Using Gates drills, the coronal segment of the root canal is progressively widened.

C Gates drills sizes #1 and #2 are used with EDTA rinses to approach the larger instrument fragment.

D/E Using an ultrasonic tip, the instrument fragment is loosened or circumnavigated.

F After rinsing with citric acid, a calcium hydroxide dressing is placed and left *in situ* for four weeks.

G Radiograph of the final results after retreatment. The smaller instrument fragment could not be removed and it was simply circumnavigated during reinstrumentation.

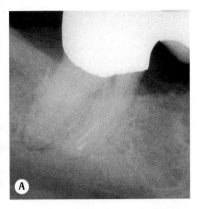

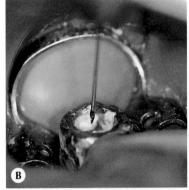

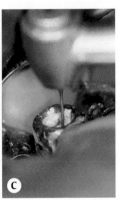

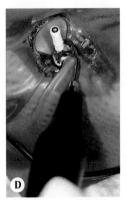

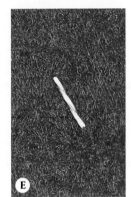

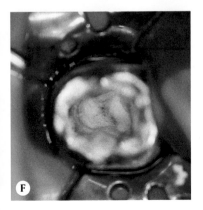

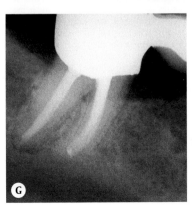

Perforations represent the second most common reason for endodontic failure. The most favorable chance for success resides with immediate closure of the perforation, and the chances increase with increasing distance from the apex:

- perforations in the **coronal third** can be treated and closed using an orthograde approach
- in the **middle third,** surgical exposure of the perforation is usually indicated
- in the **apical third,** apicoectomy or root amputation or tooth hemisection must be performed.

Diagnosis of a **perforation** of the root is performed by inserting a **paper point** into the dried root canal. Blood on the tip of the paper point indicates overinstrumentation; blood on side indicates a lateral perforation or a root fissure. The precise location of the perforation can be ascertained using the **electronic length measurement device** after any hemorrhage has been stilled. After coronal fixation of a prebent K file with IRM cement, a **radiograph** is used to check the distance from a fixed reference point, and the direction of the notch on the rubber stop will indicate the three-dimensional position.

After localizing the perforation, denatured collagen (quantity determined by position and size of the perforation) is pressed into the lateral periodontal tissues via a plugger; this is done to create a buttress. Then a thin Hedström file is inserted into the primary canal and left *in situ;* using a graduated plugger, well-mixed MTA cement (ProRoot, Dentsply) is applied in small portions into the perforation canal up to the buttress; this serves to effectively close the perforation site.

If copious bleeding into the root canal occurs from the perforation site, the hemorrhage must be stilled before any additional treatment. This can be accomplished by carefully injecting **calcium hydroxide** into the perforation site and the primary canal using a syringe. Five minutes later, the calcium hydroxide is rinsed out using sodium hypochlorite solution. This procedure is repeated three or four times, until the bleeding is stopped. If, despite these efforts, adequate

hemostasis is not achieved, a dressing consisting of $Ca(OH)_2$ is placed into the canal and left there for seven days. Other choices of materials such as calcium sulfate or MTA may also be used. Ferrous sulfate must never be employed, because it can leave behind a blood coagulum that will enhance bacterial proliferation on the osseous wall.

In comparison to other hemostatic agents, tissue reaction to the **collagen sponge** is acceptable, thanks to complete resorption of the material and new bone formation (in experimental defects). Perforations that are sealed using freeze-dried bone exhibit the formation of a connective tissue capsule six months later.

In addition, **mineral trioxide** (MTA) induces short-term and long-term synthesis of new osteoid cementum, with significantly better reaction compared with all other closure materials. Application is by means of a teflon-coated plugger. MTA is a nonresorbable material.

Calcium sulfate (Capset, Lifecore Biomaterials, Chaska) is indicated not only as a barrier but also as a hemostatic agent. It provides a tamponade effect and closes the vascular channels once it has set. Capset is sufficiently biocompatible, and is resorbed in two to four weeks. It is applied into the root defect using a syringe; it hardens rapidly and can be finished down using an ultrasonic finisher (UFI, Dentsply). In a moist field of operation, calcium sulfate is the substance of choice.

Case Presentation

A–C The radiograph depicts a perforation of the root, which had been filled with a cement. The primary canal had not been instrumented beyond the perforation. After opening coronally, hemorrhage was stilled and the location of the perforation was determined.

D–F A buttress is formed over the perforation site using resorbable collagen forced into the periapical bone, and MTA or SuperEBA is placed using a graduated plugger.

G–I Before treatment of the perforation itself, the apical primary canal is located using a Hedström file; it is instrumented, rinsed, and filled. Thereafter, the perforation is closed using MTA.

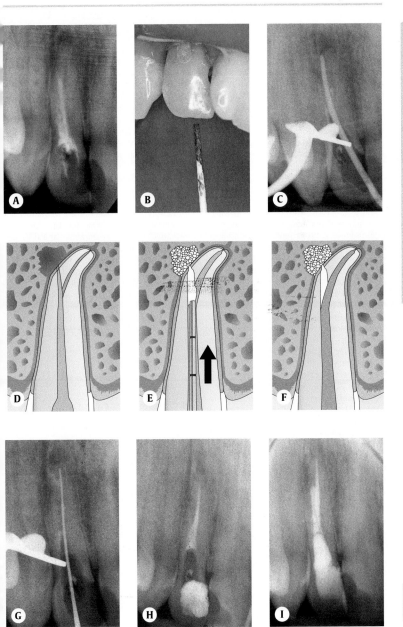

Perforations at or near the bifurcation occur in 3–10% of cases. The prognosis is dependent upon prevention and the treatment of a possible bacterial infection. With aseptic technique and immediate closure, the success rate is very high.

Root perforations at the height of the alveolar crest may communicate with periodontal pockets, and therefore have a low success rate. Orthograde canal fillings are unsatisfactory; surgical intervention is recommended.

Perforations often occur in the coronal root segment during preparation of the access cavity, during the search for obliterated canals, or during preparation of the tooth to receive an endodontic post build-up. Clinical evidence of such perforations includes blood on the paper point, unexpected pain upon probing within the canal, and persistent copious hemorrhage.

In order to avoid perforations, the clinician must use the diagnostic radiograph to measure the distance to the pulpal floor **before** preparation of the access cavity. The bleeding that occurs after perforation can usually be stopped with a sterile cotton pellet, or the pellet can be first soaked in epinephrine (1:50 000). Then collagen is forced through the perforation into the surrounding bone; it also serves to staunch hemorrhage. Other materials may also be employed: freeze-dried bone, calcium sulfate (Capset), or MTA (ProRoot).

If the perforation defect can be directly visualized (e.g., loupes, surgical microscope), it is lightly reinstrumented with an ultrasonic finisher (UF1-1C through 4C, Dentsply) so that the definitive filling material can be subsequently applied easily and with control.

The use of collagen (e.g., Collacote, Sulger Dental, Carlsbad) provides good hemostasis. It is biocompatible, supports new tissue growth, is completely resorbed within ca. 10–14 days, and can be left in the osseous wound. Depending upon the location and size of the defect, small pieces of collagen are applied with a teflon-coated plugger into and onto the perforation until a visible barrier is created at the floor of the cavity. Bleeding should stop in two ot five minutes. This **collagen barrier** prevents the penetration of sealing agents that have not yet set. Final closure and sealing is performed using a nonresorbable, impermeable, and biocompatible material such as SuperEBA cement (Bosworth, Skogie), calcium phosphate cement, or MTA.

The endodontic treatment can now be completed; the closure substance is appraised and enhanced as necessary, and the floor of the cavity is covered with a glass ionomer cement. The final procedure is definitive closure of the trepanation opening, using an appropriate adhesive filling material, which also seals the occlusal surface.

Perforations in the coronal third of the root canal should be closed and sealed with calcium sulfate whenever possible, because this is the only material that both sets rapidly and does not absorb moisture during the adhesive process. This is particularly important in cases where the definitive filling and restoration will employ adhesive restorative materials.

Perforations coronal to the gingival margin can be simply filled using a tooth-colored restorative material; perforations apical to the gingival margin may require additional surgical treatment if the perforation is inaccessible or very large, as well as in cases of massive of overfilling. After exposing the defect via soft tissue flap reflection with or without osteotomy, the perforation opening is closed with IRM or SuperEBA cement; the root surfaces are planed and a resorbable membrane is employed as necessary.

Case Presentation

A A perforation occurred during the search for the distobuccal canal.

B The perforation canal that was believed to be the distobuccal canal exhibited no hemorrhage; the actual canal orifice was revealed and exposed using ultrasonics.

C Using electronic length measurements, the actual canal is prepared from the coronal aspect.

D Optical check of the perforation and of the distobuccal canal orifice, as well as hemostasis.

E The distobuccal canal is filled and sealed using a gutta percha point, and the perforation is treated.

F Radiographic view of the endodontic treatment.

G/H Application of collagen over the perforation, and subsequent coverage with MTA.

I Radiograph taken four years later.

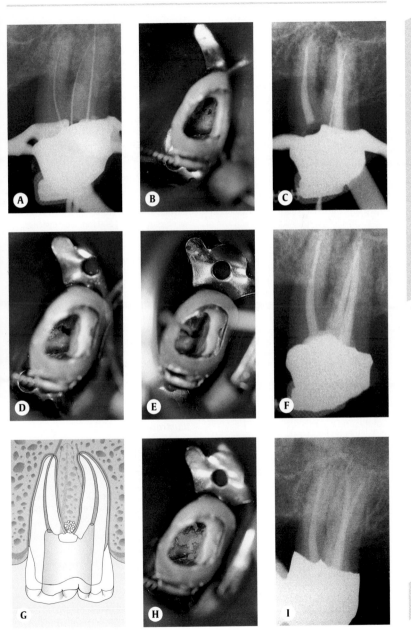

Endodontic surgery is categorized as:
• incision and drainage
• periradicular and corrective surgery
• extraction and reimplantation.

During the **apicoectomy** procedure, sections of the root that are incompletely instrumented and filled are removed. The procedure simplifies apical preparation for the placement of a retrograde filling material that seals the apical interface of the root canal and the periapical tissues.

Apicoectomy is **indicated** if conventional endodontic treatment has failed, or if retreatment fails or is not indicated but the tooth must be maintained. Even a highly experienced clinician must think long, hard, and critically when faced with surgical retreatment of an endodontically elicited periapical lesion. Demanding consideration is the fact that the procedure is a quite invasive one, with surgical limitations. The required sacrifice of tooth hard structure may be unacceptable, and there exist additional potential complications such as vertical fracture and perforation. Surgical removal of a large segment of the root brings with it complete loss of the apical constriction; this permits ingress of bacterial metabolic products into the periapical tissues via numerous severed dentinal tubuli.

Nevertheless, within a **narrow range of indications** and critical evaluation of potential risks, the apicoectomy procedure remains as a valuable adjunct to conservative endodontics and orthograde retreatment when the latter have failed.

In general, there are **four primary indications**:
• defective conservative endodontic treatment
• enlargement or persistence of a periapical radiolucency
• anatomic aberrations
• errors during canal instrumentation, e.g., perforations, instrument fracture, overfilling or underfilling of the canal, and appearance or persistence of clinical symptoms.

If an apical radiolucency persists following conventional endodontic treatment, or if orthograde retreatment is impractical, the alternative is periapical surgery. Many of the previously accepted indications for apicoectomy are viewed with some hesitation today, because the introduction of new materials, techniques and above all the surgical microscope have provided new possibilities for **nonsurgical** retreatment. When formulating a definitive indication for surgery, clinical symptoms such as pain, swelling and fistula formation, periapical radiolucency, and the quality of the root canal filling must be considered, as well as the patient's dental and medical histories.

Surgical endodontics has undergone fundamental changes: The **surgical microscope** has improved diagnosis and made possible new avenues for root canal preparation and closure of apical ramifications and/or lateral perforations. The microscope should provide a five-stage magnification from 4–25× magnification, must provide a 180° moveable binocular, as well as an objective with a 200 mm focal distance.

When one contemplates surgery, the most fundamental visual and radiographic examination of the tooth and its adjacent structures remain as essential prerequisites. The soft tissues must be examined for swelling, fistula formation, and crepitus. In addition, the surgical **approach** must be determined. The radiograph must provide information concerning spatial relationships to adjacent roots and the proximity of important anatomic structures such as the mental foramen, inferior alveolar nerve or the maxillary sinuses. When treating premolars and molars, the spatial relationship of the roots must be clearly determined using two radiographs taken with different projection angles.

Illustrations

A Complete microsurgical instrumentarium: This includes the microprobe VA7, spatula VA9–14, microspoon excavator VA16, and carver VA20.

B Microsurgical scalpel CK1-5 (EIE) with bilateral cutting edges that can be inserted into a round holder (Aesculap BB46).

C Micromirrors and mouth mirror in comparison.

D Ultrasonic handpiece for retrograde preparation with retropreparation tips.

E Diamond-coated retrotips 15 RD/LD.

F S13LD for the left maxilla/right mandible, and S13RD for the right maxilla/left mandible.

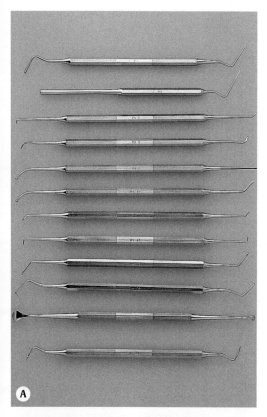

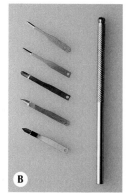

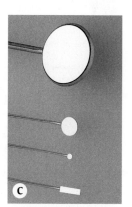

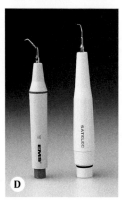

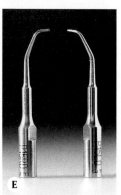

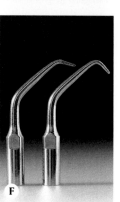

The goal of **microsurgical treatment** is complete healing and long-term freedom from symptoms. In the arena of **soft tissue management**, healthy and diseased marginal tissue are distinguished:

- with healthy tissue, one can expect rapid healing with maintenance of the gingival niveau vis-à-vis the crown margin.
- with healing by secondary intention, gingival recession is to be expected.

The incision is performed with a microscalpel held in a round handle (Aesculap BB46). The minimal magnification to control the incision line under the surgical microscope is 4–8×. Maintenance of the interdental papillae deserves special attention. The vertical releasing incisions should be extended far enough apically to ensure minimal tension on the soft tissue flap.

Three **types of mucoperiosteal flaps** are acknowledged:

- The **"triangular flap"** is easy to prepare and ensures good vascular supply; however, it does not provide optimum access. It is indicated mostly for use in cases of perforation.
- The "triangular flap" can be modified into a **"rectangular flap,"** which permits good mobilization of the soft tissues. A possible disadvantage is subsequent gingival recession.
- Following a horizontal incision and bilateral vertical releasing incision, the **Ochsenbein–Luebke flap** courses within the attached gingiva. A very narrow zone of attached gingiva results, and osseous resorption may extend to the level of the horizontal incision.

The suture material of choice is 7/0 polypropylene, which must be removed three to five days later.

It is recommended that the patient ingest 800 mg of ibuprofen one-half hour before the surgery, to reduce postoperative pain and inflammatory reactions. Precise localization of the field of operation can be difficult if the osseous wall is not perforated by the lesion. The root length is measured radiographically from the cementoenamel junction. The expanse of the osseous opening should be as small as possible. At 10–16× magnification, apical tooth structures and bone can be clearly differentiated. At 10–25× magnification the etiology of the failure can usually be identified: multiple apical or lateral foramina, and additional canals that are not visible in the radiograph, as well as overfilling or underfilling of the canal, and root fractures.

Following localization of the roots, all granulation tissue is removed to provide better observation of the root anatomy. For hemostasis, ferrous sulfate solution (Cuttrol) is used in small osseous defects; adrenalin-soaked cotton pellets (1:50 000) or resorbable cellulose sponge, as well as calcium sulfate in larger osseous defects.

The expanse of osseous **resection** and the angle of resection remain the subject of controversial discussion. Recommendations for the angle of root resection vary between 30 and 90° to the long axis of the tooth. A steep angulation, however, opens too many dentinal tubuli, bringing with it the danger of a failure. The **angle of resection** is dependent upon the inclination and dilaceration of the root, the osseous thickness, the tooth type, and its position in the alveolus.

During the apicoectomy procedure, the angle of resection should be as near as possible perpendicular to the long axis of the tooth; in some cases, however, access and vision demand less of an angle. At 16–20× magnification and with use of a micromirror, resection and angle can be held to a minimum.

Illustrations

A–C Preparation of a submarginal, right-angle flap (Ochsenbein–Luebke).

D–F Preparation of a triangular flap, with an intrasulcular and one vertical incision; with a second vertical incision, the flap can be expanded into a rectangular flap.

G A length of 3 mm was excised from the root tip; this ensures that 90 % of all apical ramifications and lateral canals are removed.

H For hemostasis, cotton pellets are tamponated into the osseous defect; only the first pellet is saturated with a hemostatic agent.

I After three minutes, the final pellet is left in situ, and the root canal is prepared and filled from the retrograde approach. Finally the pellet is removed.

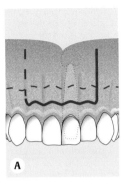

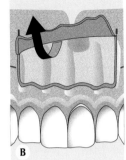

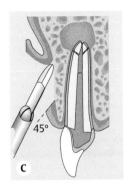

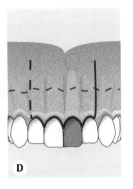

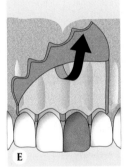

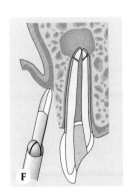

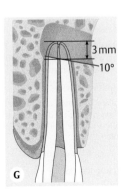

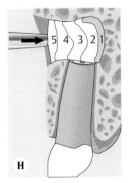

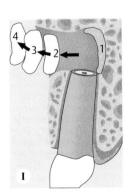

Once the osseous resection cavity has been tamponated and the bleeding stopped, the root surface is carefully examined using a **micromirror** CX-1 at 15–25× magnification.

Staining the surface with **methylene blue** (Canal Blue, VDW) brings anatomic structures into better visual prominence. Following removal of excess stain using sterile NaCl solution, it is easier to inspect the periodontal ligament and other apical structures such as canal orifices, isthmus, C-shaped canals, fracture lines and canal ramifications, as well as insufficient root canal filling material and extruded gutta percha. This is of decisive importance for treatment success. Traditionally the resection surface was examined using a fine explorer and the naked eye; however, without a surgical microscope fine structures such as isthmus tissue, fracture lines, or additional smaller canals are unlikely to be detected.

One of the most frequent causes for failure in endodontic and microsurgical therapy is poor adaptation of the root canal filling material. The success rate for surgical endodontic treatment of posterior teeth is 44–73%, while with similar treatment of anterior teeth the figure is 85–90%. It is relatively easy to resect the root tip of the mesiobuccal root of maxillary first molars. Nevertheless, the success rate was poorer when compared with mandibular molars even though the latter are more difficult to treat. In addition to technical problems, possible causes for this fact include above all untreated canals and failure to detect/locate the canal isthmus, which represents a corridor, a lateral connection, or anastomosis of two separate root canals. This isthmus can contain necrotic or infected pulpal tissue. Only 15% of anterior teeth have a single isthmus, and 20% of distal mandibular roots, but 60% of maxillary first molars.

Preparation is performed using an **ultrasonic retrotip**, which may also be diamond-coated. Subsequent observation at 16× magnification will depict whether canals and isthmus are clean and appropriately prepared, and whether the retrograde preparation has elicited any microfractures; the latter would necessitate further resection. The advantage of ultrasonic preparation is that it is not only gentler to the hard structure, but also permits exact preparation to a precisely determined

depth of 3 mm. An osteotomy opening of only 5 mm or less is adequate, because the ultrasonic tips are only 3 mm long and the shaft is graceful. This combination leads to more rapid and better healing of the osteotomy wound.

Drying of the rinsed retropreparation is accomplished with paper points and the **Stropko-Irrigator** (EIE) with a microtip.

Retrograde closure of the root canal is accomplished using **SuperEBA cement** (Bosworth), or well-mixed **Diaket**, or with **MTA cement**. For use of SuperEBA, a small amount of liquid is mixed on a glass slab with abundant powder until the surface takes on a moist shine. The mixture is rolled into a 2–3 mm long and 1 mm thick cone, and inserted into the preparation. The setting reaction can be accelerated by applying a cotton pellet that has been dipped into hot water. The resection surface is smoothed using a carbide finishing bur.

The mucoperiosteal flaps are adapted using 7/0 sutures. Smooth, solid suture material (Supramid) helps to inhibit plaque accumulation. In order to achieve optimum regeneration, suture removal should be performed three to five days postoperatively.

Case Presentation

A–C Failed endodontic treatment of maxillary anterior tooth 12, exhibiting an enlarging periapical lesion (one year after filling).

D After staining, the ultrasonic tip CT-1 is used for preparation to a depth of 3 mm, thereafter additional preparation using the CT-5.

E Applying the SuperEBA cement.

F The filling is compacted using a burnisher, and a periodontal curette is used to remove the excess; finally a carbide finishing bur is used for smoothing.

G Preoperative: periapical lesion with fistula.

H Postoperative: retrograde closure

I Control radiograph taken one year later exhibits osseous regeneration.

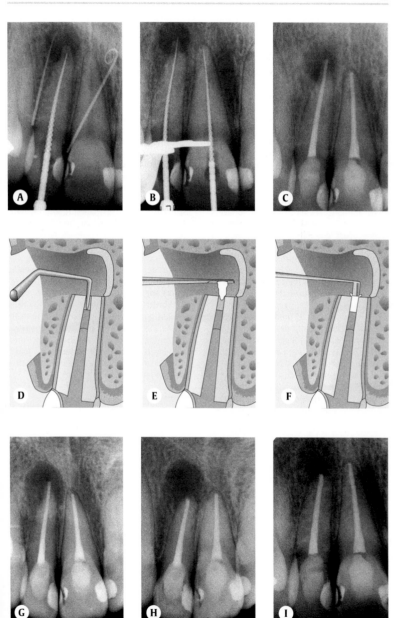

The **thermocatalytic method** of bleaching involves the use of hydrogen peroxide (H_2O_2) solution that is brought into contact with the tooth surfaces using loosely woven gauze strips. Heat is then applied using special lamps or thermostatically controlled heat rods; the temperature must not exceed 55°C. Before any bleaching of vital teeth, a brief superficial etching with phosphoric acid is recommended.

Professional dental prophylaxis removes the pellicle as well as any superficial stains. The enamel is thoroughly cleaned, the gingiva is coated with Vaseline to prevent any soft tissue irritation, and an extrastrong rubber dam is applied. In cases exhibiting heavy or tenacious staining, the entire tooth surface is etched for 10 seconds. Cotton pellets are pulled apart and placed loosely upon the tooth surface, then 30% hydrogen peroxide is applied dropwise and heated for two minutes with a special heating rod (Touch'n'Heat). The bleaching solution is then reapplied and the procedure is performed three to five times during a single appointment.

The **walking bleach method** can only be used on endodontically treated teeth. An inadequate root canal filling must first be retreated, and sealed using a 2 mm thick layer of glass ionomer cement. Subsequently, a mixture of hydrogen peroxide and sodium perborate is placed into the cavity and any excessive fluid is removed using paper points. The walking bleach solution is then covered with Cavit or GIZ, and then changed at two-to-seven-day intervals. Finally, Calxyl dressing is placed for 10 days and covered with Cavit. In one study, it was shown that the bleaching solutions lose effectiveness with time even when properly stored. Fresh sodium perborate and H_2O_2 provide lightening of tooth color in 93% of patients; on the other hand, a mixture of fresh sodium perborate and H_2O_2 that had been stored for one year provided effective bleaching in only 73% of patients. Sodium perborate mixed with water bleached only 55% of stained tooth crowns. Extreme care is indicated when using this bleaching procedure, because external resorptions are possible.

For the **vital bleaching** of individual teeth or entire arch segments, a 10% carbamide peroxide gel in a **night guard** can be used.

Depending upon the patient's cooperation, lightening of the tooth crown color may be observed as early as two to three weeks later, and is complete after five to six weeks. An at-home bleaching technique is indicated for the removal of external (extrinsic) stains such as coffee, tea or tobacco. In combination with other bleaching techniques, even internal (intrinsic) stains can be successfully removed.

To initiate the bleaching procedure, the tooth surfaces are thoroughly cleaned, and a plaster model is fabricated from an alginate impression. In order to prevent soft tissue irritation, the labial surfaces of the teeth to be bleached are blocked with acrylic resin at a distance of 0.5 mm from the gingival margin. Afterwards a thin, permanently soft, vacuum-formed tray is prepared. At the next appointment, the tray is tried in, and the patient is instructed concerning wearing the device. Following toothbrushing in the evening, the patient applies a small amount of bleaching gel into the tray, inserts it slowly and then removes any excess with a cotton swab or the toothbrush. If the bleaching tray is only used at night, a duration of treatment of four to six weeks will be necessary. If the tray is worn also during the day and the bleaching solution is changed every two to three hours, maximum bleaching effect can be achieved after seven to ten days.

Case Presentation

A–C Maxillary incisor exhibiting an inadequate root canal filling; this must be retreated and covered with GIZ before bleaching treatment.

D Appearance of the crown before bleaching.

E Thermocatalytic bleaching with 30% hydrogen peroxide, activated by heat.

F Appearance after 5× external bleaching.

G Placement of the mixed walking bleach paste (sodium perborate, plus 3% H_2O_2).

H Final filling with calcium hydroxide.

I Appearance six weeks later.

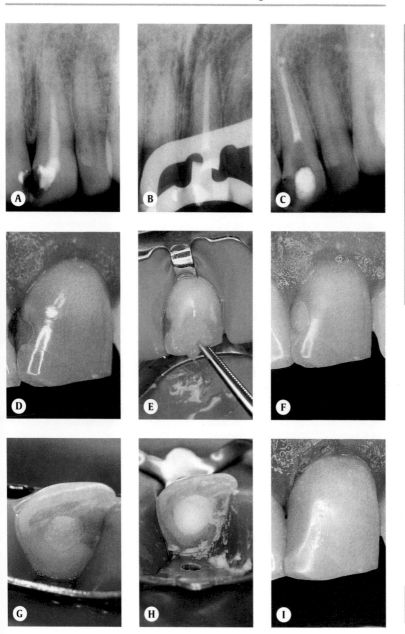

Definitive **restoration of the crown** is an integral component of endodontic therapy. Even obturated root canals can become recontaminated with microorganisms, if:

- restoration of the crown is performed too late
- the temporary filing is not impermeable between appointments
- the restoration or the tooth fractures
- the apical segment of the root canal filling is too short (<3 mm) following preparation of the master gutta percha point.

In a study of 742 root canal fillings, the 46% exhibiting poor success rate had both poor coronal restorations as well as insufficient root canal fillings. A poor restoration in combination with a good root canal filling led to success in 71% of cases. Endodontic treatment success was observed in 79% of patients with a good coronal restoration but a poor root canal treatment, and in 86% with both a good restoration and impermeable apical closure. As demonstrated by this study, the quality of the coronal restoration is just as important as the quality of the root canal filling in terms of overall success.

In addition, the choice of **material** for definitive restoration of the **crown** has a significant influence on overall success. In a two-year study, endodontically treated teeth restored with a full crown exhibited the highest success rate (over 70%); on the other hand, temporary restoration with IRM cement (57%) as well as amalgam restorations (51%) were clearly poorer in terms of long-term success.

If, following endodontic treatment, the access cavity is not impermeably closed, bacteria can penetrate any unfilled portions of the root canal within 48 hours. Even canals with excellent, impermeable root canal fillings become contaminated with bacteria after four to 48 days if the trepanation opening and coronal cavity remain unfilled. On the other hand, if the access cavity is impermeably closed, virtually no bacterial penetration will occur.

Bacterial endotoxins can also penetrate the root canal filling within three weeks; however, if the coronal closure is impermeable, no endotoxins can be detected in the canal.

Fracture of endodontically treated teeth is often explained by the reduced physical characteristics of the dentin. However, dentin from vital teeth or endodontically treated exhibit **no** differences in strength or resistance. Nevertheless, both the shape and form of the access cavity as well as the final restoration will influence the danger of fracture. Following MO preparations, the load-bearing capacity was 81% of normal, and after MOD preparation, only 61%.

Removal of the pulp chamber roof and any ledges significantly reduces the load-bearing capacity. Molars normally fracture with a load of 341 kg; an MOD preparation reduced this to 222 kg. In teeth with an endodontic access cavity and an MOD preparation, fracture occurred after only a 121 kg load.

The definitive restoration of endodontically treated teeth using amalgam leads to unsatisfactory results over the long term. Teeth with an MOD restoration exhibit fractures more frequently than teeth with intact marginal ridges. Thirty percent of the maxillary and 40% of mandibular premolars remained intact at the end of the period of observation. Teeth with only an MO restoration had a clearly better long-term success rate (80%).

Despite these statistics, however, an MOD restoration with amalgam reduces the danger of fracture and increases the rigidity from 61 to 82%; on the other hand, this figure is increased to 125% through use of a cast partial crown "capping the cusps." Endodontically treated posterior teeth must be restored with a **partial crown**, "**capping the cusps**" in order to guarantee long-term protection against tooth fracture.

Case Presentation

A Mandibular molar exhibiting periapical radiolucency.

B–D Instrumentation and root canal filling after a four-week Ca(OH)$_2$ temporary dressing.

E/F Immediately thereafter, the tooth crown was built-up and prepared for definitive restoration with a new partial crown, an impression was taken and a temporary crown was seated. Only one week later, the definitive restoration was seated. Occlusal view of the partial crown, which protects the tooth from overloading and fracture.

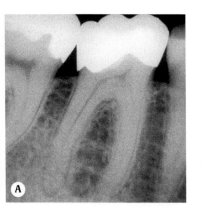

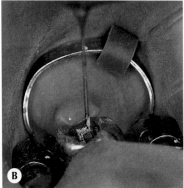

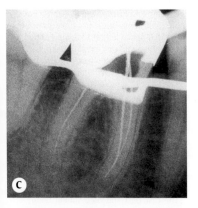

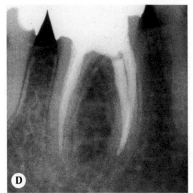

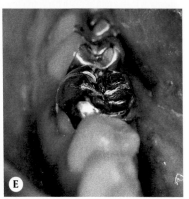

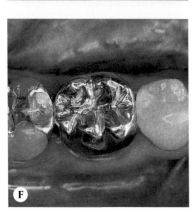

The **type of restoration** following endodontic treatment will depend upon the amount of remaining tooth hard structure and upon the forces that the restored tooth must absorb/resist. **Anterior teeth** can be easily restored with an acrylic filling if the access defect is not too large. The frequency of fracture of anterior teeth is only 2% less if a full crown restoration is used. In contrast, non-crowned **posterior teeth** are clearly much more susceptible to fracture (38–48%) compared with teeth restored with full crown restorations (10% for premolars and 5% for molars).

Posts cemented into the root canal might be expected to lead to some strengthening of the weakened root. However, laboratory investigations have demonstrated that the preparation of the canal to receive a post leads to additional weakening of the tooth hard substance, and that seating the post does not increase the resistance of the tooth vis-à-vis its condition before preparation. **Posts** anchored in the root canal do **not** serve to **strengthen** the root; the post serves only to provide additional retention for the build-up and the replacement crown.

The highest resistance to fracture is provided by the cast build-up system ("post and core"). Prefabricated posts with a composite resin build-up fracture with only half of the loading, and were only insignificantly stronger than a 3 mm adhesive composite build-up within the canal without any post.

Planning for a cast post and core demands consideration for adequate length. The retention of the post in these canals will be increased by almost 50% if the length is increased from 5–8 mm. The **length of the post in the canal** should:

- be ca. two-thirds of the entire canal length
- correspond to the tooth's crown length
- correspond to one-half of the root length supported by alveolar bone.

Parallel-wall posts exhibit a 2–4× better retention than conically shaped posts. In addition, the forces are better transferred to the canal walls and the danger of fracture is lower. **Conical post systems** are indicated only in mandibular anterior teeth of small diameter. Indicated here are cast post systems exclusively, which exhibit the highest resistance values. The use of castable parapost systems brings with it the danger of fracture within the post system itself.

The definitive **cast post and core** is cemented at the next appointment. Invitro studies showed that the best sealing was achieved with cyanoacrylate cement, followed by polycarboxylate cement and an acrylic cement after dentin etching. The poorest sealing was exhibited by phosphate cement. If eugenol-containing sealer is used, the canal dentin must be conditioned with citric acid and rinsed with ethanol before cementation.

There exists no principal difference between the preparation for a post build-up at the same appointment after root canal filling, or at a subsequent appointment. Regardless of whether the gutta percha is removed mechanically or thermally, the impermeability of the remaining root canal filling of 4 mm is equally good. Clinical investigations have shown that a minimal apical length of 3 mm is required. With a remaining root canal filling distance of 5 mm, the failure rate was 10%, but almost 30% with a 2 mm remaining root canal filling.

The successful function of a tooth following endodontic treatment will be determined to a great degree by the expanse of the remaining tooth structure. A full crown restoration that encompasses remaining tooth structure at the cervical region elevates the resistance of an endodontically treated tooth, independent of the presence of a post build-up. The crown margin should reside at least 1 mm into dentin.

The cast post and core should bodily encompass at least 2 mm of tooth hard structure at the margin (**Ferrule effect**). This will double the fracture resistance.

Case Presentation

A/B Symptom-free molar exhibits an inadequate amalgam restoration.

C/D The cast post and core is fabricated; polishing the post reduces its retention.

E Cast crowns elevate the success rate to 97%.

F/G The post and core, following conditioning of the dentin, as well as the definitive crown are seated using an acrylic-based cement.

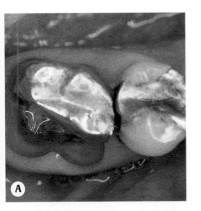

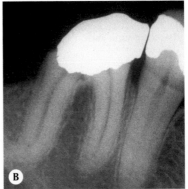

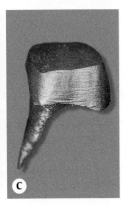

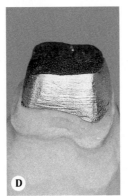

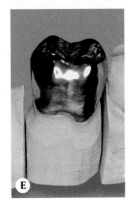

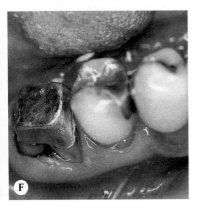

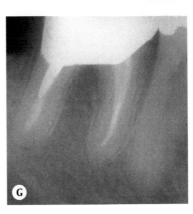

A **post build-up** consists of three elements:
- the build-up itself (which requires replacement of coronal tooth hard substance for the subsequent anchoring of a definitive coronal restoration)
- the root canal post (retention for the build-up)
- material for permanent retention within the endodontically treated tooth.

The definitive and permanent restoration of the tooth following completed endodontic treatment should be undertaken **as soon as possible** because of the risk of reinfection.

As a general rule, the length of the post influences retention more than its diameter. Post build-ups seated directly with dentin-adhesive cements are much more tissue friendly. Undercut areas and thin dentin walls can be adhesively supported and used as additional retentive surfaces.

Build-up posts for use in root canals can be categorized according to the material, the method of fabrication (individual, partially or completely prefabricated), the shape (conical, cylindrical), or the surface structure (smooth, rough, or with threads). The material must be biologically inert, exhibit a high resistance to breakage, and be perfectly adaptable. Modern, metal-free post systems consist of either high-resistant ceramics (e.g., zirconium oxide), or composite materials, strengthened by carbon or glass fibers. In comparison to metal posts, these posts exhibit a dentin-like biomechanical property and have the advantage that they can be relatively easily removed if necessary.

Individual (prefabricated) post systems are particularly indicated for the restoration of severely broken down teeth. Threaded posts with cylindrical geometry achieve the highest retention values, but they also cause higher concentrations of tension within the canal. Posts exhibiting cylindrical geometry are preferred to conical posts because of their better retention if the post is shorter than the crown. Passive, conical posts correspond best to the root canal anatomy; the elevated risk of loss of retention is reduced by the adhesive seating and the retentive surface structure. The canal walls and the access cavity are conditioned for 20 seconds with 37% phosphoric acid, and then sprayed with water, and the canal is then rinsed with alcohol and carefully dried with air. Using a 0.8-mm one-time applicator (Brush XS), the bonding material is applied in the canal and to the post; excess material is removed using a paper point. The fine-particle hybrid adhesive composite (Compolute Applikap, ESPE) is gently rotated into the canal using a Lentulo spiral, the post is then painted with the adhesive and slowly inserted into the canal.

The **adhesive technique** stabilizes the coronoradicular complex. The subsequent coronal build-up is performed using a composite resin system. Prefabricated crown shells (Forms-to-Fit or Frasaco) are filled with composite resin and then light hardened. In a recently published study (Mezzomo et al. 2003), carbon composite posts seated with zinc phosphate cement or with a resin cement (C&B), exhibited equally high resistance values (106.5–107.1) if they were surrounded by a 2 mm wide cervical dentin ferrule. Without this dentin ring, the loading limit was only 71.3 to 84 kg. The stability of the post build-up is significantly increased when a minimally 2 mm wide dentin margin (**ferrule**) remains apical to the build-up, and which is subsequently encompassed by the definitive crown.

Case Presentation

A/B Inadequate root canal filling, apical radiolucency, and fractured crown.

C After dissolving with eucalyptol, the filling was removed and the canal reinstrumented.

D During the same appointment, the canals were filled and a prefabricated temporary crown was seated.

E Distally, the preparation extended to the depth of the crown.

F/G The metal post build-up was cemented to place, and the crown was formed using composite resin.

H/I After a periodontal crown lengthening procedure to achieve a 2 mm wide ferrule effect, the definitive crown was seated using adhesive cement.

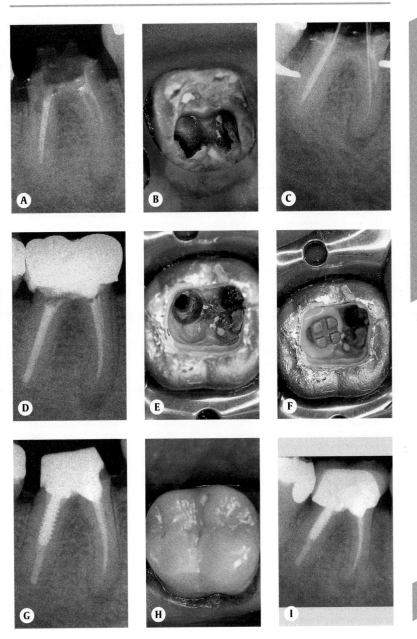

The dentin of endodontically treated teeth does not exhibit any reduced load-bearing capacity. Endodontic treatment changes the **mechanical characteristics of the tooth** only insignificantly. In one study, 23 teeth that had been endodontically treated 10 years previously and an equal number of vital teeth from the same patients were tested with regard to biomechanical properties. Endodontically treated teeth fractured under a load of 611 N, and vital teeth at 574 N. Nevertheless, the loss of hard tooth structure can negatively influence mechanical characteristics. Given this fact, the **quantity** of dentin remaining within the tooth crown determines to a great degree the load-bearing capacity of an endodontically treated and restored tooth.

The most important consideration for prevention of tooth fracture is not the post design, but rather the definitive crown restoration. The majority of studies of frequency of fracture of post-restored roots were performed without any coronal restoration. The reported differences between and among the individual post systems disappear if a crown is seated. The fracture frequency is much more dependent upon the type of coronal restoration that to the post. The failure rate for parallel-wall posts and crowned teeth is only 6.5% after 10 years. The six-year success rate with a composite resin build-up is 81%, and that for cast post and core, 91%. The long-term behavior and success of glass-fiber or carbon-reinforced build-ups have not yet been reported; only studies up to 32 months are available and the results are promising, without failures.

As a general rule, therefore, a post should only be inserted if it is absolutely required by the prosthetic reconstruction of the tooth due to lack of coronal hard tissue. Fracture resistance before and/or after seating a post build-up is not different, but predrilling the tooth to receive a post does lead to further weakening of the treated tooth.

Because of the lack of clinical studies to provide clear evidence of superior treatment concepts, currently various treatment methods are favored; the dentist is confronted with a panoply of therapy alternatives that can scarcely be understood. In the literature, the length of time between endodontic and restorative therapy is given as six months, but there is not one single study to support or prove this statement! On the other hand, numerous studies recommend the **immediate definitive treatment** in order to avoid any coronal permeabilities. Even the existence of a periapical lesion is not a contraindication for definitive restoration! If a periapical radiolucency shows signs of enlarging, apicoectomy is the treatment of choice. Immediate root tip resection is associated with a lower success rate, and therefore offers only disadvantages in comparison to conventional endodontic treatment.

The **quality of the crown used to restore the tooth** is crucially important for the overall success of endodontic therapy. The success rate with high quality root canal filling and coronal restoration is 91%, but this drops to 44% with inadequate coronal restoration, despite good endodontic treatment.

The appropriate type of restorative therapy for an endodontically treated tooth depends upon the tooth type and its clinical condition. Full coverage for anterior teeth is only indicated in exceptional situations. In posterior teeth, a capping-the-cusps onlay is the treatment method of first choice. In a study of the restorative treatment of 745 endodontically treated teeth, the failure rate was 29.5% for teeth with full crowns, which was significantly better than teeth with composite resin definitive restorations (40.5%). The loss of hard structure during preparation of the tooth to receive the restoration additionally weakens the tooth. A restoration-specific risk analysis must be performed **before** endodontic treatment, and this must include evaluation of the prosthetic value of the tooth.

Case Presentation

A–C Restoration of an end-standing molar using an adhesive cemented ceramic inlay.

D/E Seating a bridge construction on endodontically treated teeth, 37–35.

F/G Maxillary end-standing tooth 18 after endodontic treatment and seating of a fixed bridge on tooth 16.

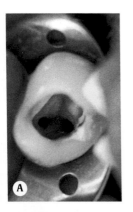

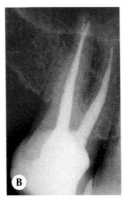

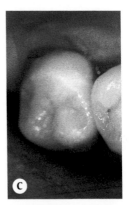

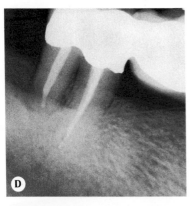

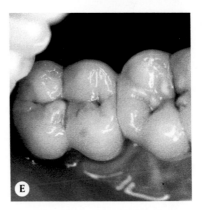

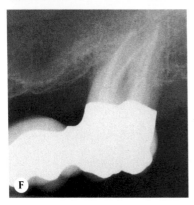

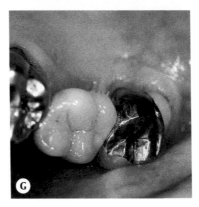

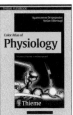
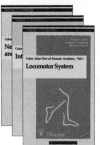
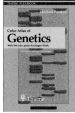
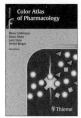
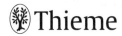